- Are you often a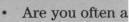
- Do you have tro
- Do you find yourself constantly worrying for no apparent reason?
- Does the stress in your life sometimes seem overwhelming?
- Do you suffer from insomnia?
- Are you worried about the side effects of prescription antianxiety drugs?

IF YOU ANSWERED YES TO ANY OF THESE QUESTIONS, READ ABOUT HOW KAVA MAY BE RIGHT FOR YOU!

"Dr. Sahelian has thoroughly reviewed the kava literature and presents the information in a practical and common sense way. *Kava: The Miracle Antianxiety Herb* is an excellent resource for consumers and health care practitioners alike who want to learn how to best make the most of this fascinating South Pacific herb."

Yadhu N. Singh, Ph.D., internationally known kava expert, and Professor of Pharmacology, College of Pharmacy, South Dakota State University, in Brookings, South Dakota.

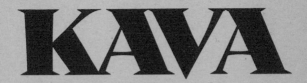

KAVA

THE MIRACLE ANTIANXIETY HERB

RAY SAHELIAN, M.D.

St. Martin's Paperbacks

KAVA

ISBN: 0-312-96788-8

Printed in the United States of America

St. Martin's Paperbacks edition/June 1998

10 9 8 7 6 5 4 3 2 1

CONTENTS

CONTENTS

ACKNOWLEDGMENTS

Lise Alschuler, N.D., is Chair of the Botanical Medicine Department at Bastyr University, Seattle, Washington.

Logan Chamberlain, Ph.D., is publisher of *Herbs for Health* magazine.

Gary Friedman imports kava from the Pacific islands and is an experienced kava user for close to three decades.

Bob Martin, D.C., is a chiropractic doctor and host on KFYI-AM 910, a radio station in Phoenix, Arizona.

Jan McBarron, M.D., is board certified in preventive medicine and practices in Columbus, Georgia.

Rob McCaleb is president and founder of Herb Research Foundation in Boulder, Colorado.

Yadhu N. Singh, Ph.D., is Professor of Pharmacology, College of Pharmacy, South Dakota State University, Brookings, South Dakota. He previously held a teaching position at the School of Pure and Applied Sciences, University of the South Pacific, in Suva (Fiji). Dr. Singh was born and raised in Fiji and has published extensive review articles regarding the traditional uses of kava.

Michael W. Smith, M.D., of the Department of Psychiatry at Harbor-UCLA, in Los Angeles, researches the psychiatric effects of herbs.

Terry Willard, Ph.D., an experienced herbalist, is president of Wild Rose College of Natural Healing in Calgary, Alberta, Canada. He started using kava in 1978.

KAVA

INTRODUCTION

Pacific islanders have relished kava's wonderful calming qualities for centuries. Over the past few years, kava has become very popular in the alternative health field. Studies during the last decade have repeatedly shown this herb to be effective in reducing anxiety, and in 1990 the Federal Board of Health in Germany approved kava for the treatment of anxiety disorders. I believe that kava is poised to become as well-known as the herbs St. John's wort and ginkgo biloba.

In order to gather the information in this book, I reviewed decades of research on kava, interviewed academic experts and users, and treated patients with this herb. I am glad to be sharing my findings about this wonderful herb that both relaxes and improves mood.

The response of the patients I recommended kava to was very positive. It's certainly not as powerful as certain pharmaceutical drugs, such as Valium and Xanax, but it doesn't have some of their side effects, such as sedation and mental slowing, either. Most patients with mild to moderate cases of anxiety respond well to the relaxing effects of this herb. Kava is bound eventually to become a solid part of the armamentarium doctors use to combat anxiety disorders.

I have used kava about once or twice a week for the past year. I believe it's important for anyone who writes about a particular supplement to try it himself or herself. I enjoy the state of relaxation and well-being that kava brings on, especially since it does not interfere with mental clarity. I find it a good way to help me relax after a particularly stressful day. I also like taking kava occasionally when attending a social event, since it enhances feelings of affability.

In addition to kava, there are a number of herbs that have been touted in traditional herbal folklore as having relaxing properties. These include chamomile, hops, passionflower, skullcap, and valerian. This book includes a critical evaluation of and the latest research on these interesting herbs.

1

TALES OF THE SOUTH PACIFIC

When we sip kava, we forget there's a class system. There are no longer Ph.D.'s, princes, preachers, nor paupers. Everyone opens up, sings, and dances together."

This was my introduction to a kava ceremony that was held at the National Nutritional Foods Association convention in Las Vegas, Nevada, in July 1997. One of the companies marketing a kava product had invited natives of Tonga (a small island in the South Pacific) to share with the attendees an actual kava ceremony. A group of curious vitamin store managers were seated in a circle on a wide piece of green artificial turf facing a group of six Tongans in native costumes. The set was decorated with small palm trees and tropical flowers, providing a Pacific island–like atmosphere. A large wooden bowl filled with a brownish liquid was placed on the green turf. A middle-aged Tongan woman with a serene smile was gently stirring this liquid with a wooden spatula. Next to her was the emcee of the ceremony, Sione Ika, a small, chubby, and jocular man, embracing a small guitar and singing delightful songs from the South Pacific. He occasionally would stop singing, stand up, and do an unusual dance with sudden movements of the arms and legs while muttering one-syllable sounds such as "umph, ah, hoo, pi, ka." Then he would sit back down and continue explaining the purpose of the kava ceremony.

"With dusk approaching, and the palm trees swaying in the wind, the villagers round up around the kava bowl. Kava, to us, is a symbol of the covenant. It is important to us in many ways—socially, culturally, and religiously. We relax, tell stories, feel good, and lose our cares in the approaching night. People with good voices, and not so good voices, share of themselves through their songs. Kava helps everyone feel part of the community and the village."

I had known about kava for many years but

had long been a skeptic. Having been trained at Thomas Jefferson Medical School, a very traditional institution in Philadelphia, I always thought that herbs were a fun distraction for many in the alternative field to play with but had no serious role in medicine. They certainly could not compete with pharmaceutical drugs. Over the years, though, I have come to respect the benefits and effectiveness that many herbal products can provide.

As I sat on the green turf, one of the Tongans offered me a cup filled with the brown liquid. He graciously bowed as he offered me the drink. It was obvious that he delighted in introducing skeptical Westerners to what South Pacific islanders had known for centuries.

I sipped from the cup, swirled the brown liquid in my mouth, and could tell that it had some active ingredient since my mouth went slightly numb. While I continued sipping, Sione proceeded, "Kava is a healthy, natural way of relaxing. We don't need television. All of the villagers sit around and tell stories. We share our thoughts and our hopes. We encourage each other. Cares and worries disappear—carried away by the warm ocean wind."

I later learned that Sione was right. Studies have shown that the kava culture of the islands is a strong factor in helping to provide better social integration among the inhabitants and deepen their sense of community (Lemert 1976). One study even found that a community-based smoking cessation program combining kava ceremonies and group pledge was successful in helping almost everyone in the village give up the tobacco habit (Groth-Marnat 1996).

After a second cup and then a third, I began to feel slightly alert yet relaxed. I also got an urge to turn to my neighbors sitting next to me and chat with them. I guess you can call this a desire to socialize. There was also a sense of peacefulness and tranquility.

The experience of that afternoon convinced me to look further into the kava story. The Tongans were kind enough to offer a plastic bag of the brown root powder, and when I returned home, I continued experimenting with it. I offered it to many friends and family members, who also reported feeling the relaxing effects of this root. In addition, I bought kava pills from a health food store and bottles of the tincture. I started recommending kava to patients as an alternative to tranquilizers.

Over the next few weeks I started noticing more and more ads in health magazines touting the promises of kava. Some of the claims and promotions were very interesting.

- What do people of Fiji, Samoa, and Tonga know about relaxation that you don't?
- Ancient mystical drink your stressed-out customers will demand.
- This natural, herbal drink relaxes muscles, calms nerves, and creates a general feeling of well-being.
- Kava is now part of a new social phenomenon as the number of kava bars grows.
- In an age where stress is a way of life, and caffeine and other stimulants are a way of getting by, it's no wonder that kavakava, the relaxing herb from the South Pacific, is today's most sought-after herbal extract.
- Kava is a relaxant and a sleep aid, able to induce a feeling of relaxation, peace, and contentment, along with a sharpening of the senses.
- The kava extract in our product is believed to reduce mild anxiety and stress, calm the mind and stabilize body temperature and reduce tension in menopausal women.

Are any of these claims true? The response from patients and my own experience certainly indicated that kava does have psychopharmacological effects. However, I wasn't completely convinced until I came across the results of a new study published in 1997 in the journal *Pharmacopsychiatry*. The title of this article was "Kava-kava extract WS 1490 versus placebo in anxiety disorders—A randomized placebo-controlled 25-week outpatient trial." Prior to this study, the longest published one was an eight-week trial. But before I explain the results of this study, let me tell you some of the history and basics of this highly cherished South Pacific plant.

2
HISTORICAL ROOTS OF KAVA

During the late 1600s, Europeans discovered the beautiful South Pacific islands which, to their surprise, were already populated. These Europeans noticed that the native inhabitants of the islands, the Polynesians, were fond of drinking a ground-up powder of the root of the kava plant. They washed the roots of the plant, sun-dried them, chopped the roots into small pieces, and then made them into a powder by pounding or crushing them. This powder was diluted with water and coconut milk. The mixture was then kneaded and strained through fiber. Traditionally, kava was also prepared by chewing the stems and roots and spitting them with copious amounts of saliva in a bowl, to which water and coconut juice were added. This is rarely done now. Instead, the kava roots are pulverized into powder with giant makeshift mortars and pestles. These are sometimes made from metal drums and car axles (Norton 1994).

Preparation of kava by chewing the root and expectorating the pulp into a communal bowl did not seem very appealing to the very first European explorers who had contact with the Pacific islanders. An etching of a welcoming ceremony involving natives and Dutch sailors in 1616 has the subheading, "They [the islanders] presented their desirable drink to our people, as a thing rare and delicate, but the sight of their brewing had quenched our thirst" (Norton 1994).

The first white men credited with recording in detail the existence of the kava plant were members of Captain James Cook's team during his first voyage to the Pacific islands in 1775. In fact, Cook may have been the first white man to try the kava drink. A few years later, the plant was given the Latin name of *Piper methysticum* (the prefix *methy* is the Greek word for "wine") (Singh 1992).

We know for certain that kava has been used by Polynesians for a long time, perhaps hundreds or thousands of years. With the aid of special instruments, archaeologists from the University of New South Wales in Kensington, Australia, have found utensil artifacts that contain kavalactones, chemicals found in kava (Hocart 1993). The researchers state, "Thus it is now possible to link unequivocally kava drinking, a major aspect of the ceremonial culture of many Pacific societies, to the archaeological record." The three islands that most commonly used kava were Fiji, Samoa, and Tonga.

The practice of drinking kava for recreational, social, and medicinal purposes gradually spread over the centuries to neighboring islands and regions, including New Zealand, Australia, New Guinea, and even all the way northeast to Hawaii. It is interesting to note that the Polynesians, just like the North American Indians, had not discovered how to ferment alcoholic beverages before initial contact with the Europeans (Singh 1992). Thus, kava was for them in many ways the equivalent to alcohol for the Europeans.

The use of psychoactive plants was common in the South Pacific (Cawte 1985). Before the Europeans introduced alcohol (their drug of choice), the Polynesians were drinking kava, the inhabitants of Melanesia were using betel, and some Aborigines in Australia used pituri. It appears that each culture found its own locally available natural substance in order to reduce tension or reach an altered state of consciousness. Dr. Yadhu Singh, an expert on kava and professor at South Dakota State University College of Pharmacy, adds, "The importance of kava in Oceania [Polynesia, Melanesia, and Micronesia] should perhaps be considered in the context that every culture has had its own intoxicants, whether they be narcotics or stimulants or both. And in spite of their great diversity, the intoxicants employed have had the same kind of social status and significance. The sociological role of kava is probably similar in many aspects to that of peyote in the case of many native or 'Indian' tribes of North America, coca leaves with peoples of the South American Andes and opium and its derivatives in the Middle or Far East. The kava custom has been so widespread throughout Oceania that it might be considered the one item in their material culture that linked together most of the peoples of Oceania."

Tom Harrison, author of *Savage Civilization* published in 1937 writes, "Kava drinkers are satisfied with kava. Without it, they need, as all people seem to, some time-changer, something to modify reality without ritual or undue expense. As long as the people stuck to kava, there was no alcohol need. As mission influence grew, kava became labeled as something heathen; it was often obliterated. So, towards the end of the last century, alcohol came into its own until it became a principal trade item through which the trader got his greatest control over the native, holding him to the necessity of pro-white produce or work, so that he might satisfy this craving. Many natives died of drink."

The Polynesians drank kava for a variety of reasons (Singh 1992).

- For ceremonial purposes—whenever dignitaries visited the islands, they were offered the drink as a gesture of goodwill. Even Pope John Paul II and Hillary Rodham Clinton were offered kava during their visits to Pacific islands.
- To resolve disagreements among themselves. Kava made them relaxed and less argumentative. This was beneficial in terms of reconciling differences among parties with conflicting agendas.
- During important meetings, thus inducing a state of calmness and cooperation.
- As a ceremonial drink before the onset of a journey.
- To celebrate births and weddings.

- During burial ceremonies.
- For social purposes during gatherings with neighbors.
- As gifts to express friendships.
- As a medicine to cure certain illnesses.

With the urbanization of many Polynesian islands, a shift occurred. Those living in cities are more likely to consume alcohol instead of kava, while in the villages, kava consumption is markedly higher than alcohol (Finau 1982). In many villages or cities, kava bars often outnumber alcohol bars, and the locals get together to sip the drink from coconut shells. In many areas, the return of kava drinking is related to the reawakening of cultural identity.

If certain members of a culture want to consume a psychoactive substance, one may wonder whether kava or alcohol is a better option in terms of safety, addiction, and overall health. There could, of course, be a lot of debate about this issue, and we currently don't know the answers. Dr. Chris Cantor, Senior Research Psychiatrist at the Australian Suicide Research and Prevention at Griffith University, remarks, "How do morbidity [illness] and mortality [death] indices associated with kava use compare with alcohol, a drug with which we are all very familiar? I put such a question to a group of taxi drivers in Fiji with whom I was sharing a bowl of kava. They responded that the key difference was 'With kava you sleep—with alcohol you fight.' On discussing this point with medical personnel in Fiji and Tonga, the message was reinforced.

"It is tempting to wonder whether society might be a more peaceful place if we eradicated alcohol and replaced it with kava; however, this is just fantasy. It is also naive to assume that the ready availability of kava might lead to a decrease in alcohol consumption" (Cantor 1997).

KAVA IN THE 1990s

Over the last two decades, kava has gained more attention in the alternative medical field. There have been countless articles written about this herb in health magazines. Dozens of vitamin and herbal companies now import or distribute kava products in a variety of dosages and combinations.

Over the past few years, kava has even caught the attention of a number of pharmaceutical companies in Germany, the United States, Japan, and France. For instance, in February of 1995, the German pharmaceutical company Dr. Willmar Schwabe GmbH reported that it would buy one hundred tons of dried kava from producers in the South Pacific to manufacture an "anti-stress" pill (Decloitre 1995).

3

IMPORTANT FACTS ABOUT KAVA

Kava is the term used for both the plant and the beverage made from it. Other common names for kava in the South Pacific include kavakava, awa, and yagona. The plant generally thrives at altitudes between four hundred and one thousand feet and is naturally found in Polynesia, Melanesia, and Micronesia. The kava plant is robust, succulent, and well branched and is generally harvested when about six to eight feet high. Under proper conditions, the plant can grow to be up to eighteen feet tall. The beverage is prepared from the root of this shrub, called the pepper plant, or *Piper methysticum*. The root has a brownish color and is ground to a powder. This brownish powder is then mixed with water or coconut milk and drunk as a beverage, without being fermented. The root is also chewed, mixing it with saliva. It is believed that saliva aids in the breakdown of the starch in the root, allowing for easier availability of the psychoactive ingredients.

There are dozens of varieties of kava plants, and the roots of each of these varieties contain a different combination or proportion of active chemicals.

WHAT'S IN KAVA?

As with any herbal medicine, a number of compounds contribute to its medicinal effects. The active compounds are mostly concentrated in the root of the plant, although the leaves and stems also contain several active compounds. The kava plant contains a variety of chemicals known as kava-pyrones or kava-lactones. Specific names for some of these kavalactones include kawain or kavain, dihydrokawain, methysticin, dihydromethysticin, and yangonin (Rasmussen 1979, Haberlein 1997). Most good-quality kava roots contain about 5 to 8 percent kavalactones.

Scientific studies attempting to evaluate the components of kava started in the late 1800s when methysticin and yangonin were isolated

Chemical Structure of Kawain

(Foster 1897). From 1914 to 1933, a German chemist named Borsche isolated two additional components from the kava plant, naming them kawain and dihydrokawain (Borsche 1933). However, it wasn't until 1966 that the German pharmacologist H. J. Meyer was able to show that the kavalactones were responsible for the psychoactive properties (Volz 1997). In the 1960s, additional chemicals in the kava plant were found, including two pigments named flavokawin A and flavokawin B. One of the side effects of excessive and prolonged kava consumption is darkening of the skin. One scientist has proposed that this skin discoloration could possibly be due to the accumulation of these pigments (Shulgin 1973). Dr. Singh reports that the cause of the skin discoloration is still unknown (personal communication).

The water-soluble extract of kava contains different compounds from the fat-soluble extract. The central nervous activity of the water-soluble extract was determined in mice to have mild pain-killing ability but did not induce sleep (Jamieson 1989). The fat-soluble extract had sleep-inducing and marked pain-killing properties. The researchers state, "The pharmacological effects of kava ingestion appear to be due to the activity of the compounds present in the fat-soluble fraction." Kavalactones are poorly soluble in water (Volz 1997). It is obvious that the method of extraction of kavalactones from the plant can influence their physiological effects.

Many of the studies done with kava used a standardized extract, called WS 1490 or Laitan, from the German pharmaceutical company Dr. Willmar Schwabe. WS 1490 is a fat-soluble extract of the kava root containing about 100 milligrams of the dry extract, which includes about 70 milligrams of kava-pyrones per capsule (Volz 1997). WS 1490 is estimated to have approximately ten times the concentration of kavalactones present in the root. The kava products you find over the counter generally provide different proportions and combinations of ingredients. Several factors influence the composition of the products. These include:

- the age of the plant when harvested
- the species of the plant
- the type of soil the plant is grown in and perhaps the altitude at which the plant is grown
- whether the extracts are mostly from the root, the stem, or the leaves of the kava plant (the majority of the products on the market use the roots)
- the method of extraction

Extracts from the root are now placed in capsules and sold as kava, or kavakava, by mail order companies, vitamin stores, pharmacies, and retail stores.

HOW DOES KAVA WORK?

Since there are a number of different compounds in the kava root, including kawain, dihydrokawain, methysticin, yangonin, and others, it is likely that extracts of kava will influence a number of areas within the brain and body.

Many users of kava notice that their muscles are relaxed. This is because certain compounds in kava have the ability to go directly to muscle tissue and reduce contraction (Singh 1983).

A study done on brain tissue showed that chemicals in kava have the ability to enter the brain (Keledjian 1988) and also have the ability to attach to a number of brain cell receptors. The addition of kavalactones to brain tissue showed them to bind differently in different brain regions. The most prominent areas that were influenced by the kava extracts were the hippocampus, amygdala, and medulla oblongata (Jussofie 1994). The hippocampus, is a large forebrain structure located between the thalamus and cortex. Two of the functions of the hippocampus relate to memory and emotions. The cerebellum (an area in the brain involved in coordination) was not influenced much. This is consistent with the clinical effects of kava ingestion: A regular dose of kava has little effect on coordination, although repeated high doses could potentially cause dizziness and muscle weakness. Kava also did not bind to the frontal cortex, an area responsible for higher thinking and analytical skills. Unlike a few other psychoactive plants, such as mushrooms and peyote, the ingestion of kava has not been reported to provide significant insights or novel ways of thinking.

This study by Dr. A. Jussofie, of the Institute

for Physiology and Chemistry at the University of Essen in Germany, also determined that one of the receptors in the brain influenced by kava extracts was GABA, which stands for gamma-aminobutyric acid. GABA receptors are influenced by a number of medicines and drugs. For instance, Valium, the best-known benzodiazepine sedative, acts on GABA receptors to make us sleepy and relaxed. Apparently kava extracts are able to influence GABA receptors in some ways similar to benzodiazepines.

Another possible mechanism of action includes blocking of the action of the brain chemical dopamine (Schelosky 1995). The influence of kava chemicals on NMDA receptors in the brain has also been recently hypothesized (Walden 1997). An additional mechanism of action may relate to certain kavalactones, particularly kavain, blocking the uptake of norepinephrine by brain cells (Seitz 1997). Recently, it has been postulated that kava compounds could influence a type of serotonin receptor identified as 5-HT1A which may be important in reducing anxiety (Walden 1997).

With time, we'll discover more receptors and areas within the brain and body that kavalactones influence. It is likely that the effects of the various kavalactones in kava have an additive, or synergistic, psychoactive effect.

ROOT VERSUS LEAF

The majority of studies on kava have been done using extracts from the root. Although the stems and leaves also do contain several types of kavalactones, less is known about their full psychoactive effect. There are claims that the kavalactones in the stem are more sedating and less euphoric, while the kavalactones from the root are more likely to cause euphoria. There is disagreement in the herbal industry regarding this particular point (*Whole Foods*, December 1997, p. 69).

4

THE STUDY THAT
CONVINCED ME

Up until 1997, only a few short-term, placebo-controlled studies on kava extract ingestion had been published in the medical literature. In 1997, Dr. Hans-Peter Volz, of the Department of Psychiatry at Jena University in Germany, and Dr. M. Kieser, a researcher with the pharmaceutical company that makes a standardized extract WS 1490 (Dr. Willmar Schwabe GmbH, Karlsruhe, Germany), published the results of the longest comprehensive human trial using extracts of kava.

Ten medical centers in the southern part of Germany participated in this study involving 101 patients (Volz 1997). This was the first long-term, placebo-controlled trial investigating the safety and effectiveness of a kava extract in patients with anxiety. These patients were given one capsule three times a day of the concentrated extract called WS 1490 containing about 100 milligrams of kava root extract, which, in turn, had about 70 milligrams of kavalactones. WS 1490 is known to contain kavain, dihydrokavain, methysticin, dihydromethysticin, yangonin, and desmethoxyyangonin (Lehmann 1996).

All 101 of these patients suffered from anxiety and tension. Many had a fear of public places (agoraphobia), social phobia, generalized anxiety disorder, and adjustment disorder with anxiety. (I discuss these conditions in Chapter 6.) Those who had significant medical or psychological problems were excluded. Several psychological tests were done initially to assess the mental status of the patients and to monitor them throughout the treatment period. These tests included the Hamilton Anxiety Scale, the Clinical Global Impression Scale, and the Adjective Mood Scale. Furthermore, blood and urine tests were carried out regularly to determine red blood cell count, white blood cell count, platelet count, liver enzymes, creatinine, proteins, and glucose.

The study lasted twenty-five weeks. At the conclusion of the study, the following results were noted:

The short-term effectiveness of kava was superior to that of placebo. Most patients had an improvement within the first two months.

The long-term effectiveness of kava was superior to that of placebo. In fact, the effectiveness of kava improved with time. The specific areas that improved included anxious mood, tension, fears, and insomnia. After twenty-four weeks, 75 percent of patients improved compared to 51 percent of those on placebo.

Patients tolerated kava well. Adverse reactions were rare. Laboratory values, including red blood cell count, white blood cell count, platelet count, liver enzymes, creatinine, proteins, and glucose, were not affected. Blood pressure and heart rate did not show any changes. More patients on placebo dropped out of the study than those on kava. This indicates that those on kava did not have any problems with its ingestion.

The researchers say, "These results support WS 1490 [kava] as a treatment alternative to tricyclic antidepressants and benzodiazepines in anxiety disorders, with proven long-term efficacy and none of the tolerance problems associated with tricyclics and benzodiazepines."

A review of the medical literature published on kava indicates a number of short-term studies that have found results consistent with this 1997 study.

Back in 1991, Dr. E. Kinzler and colleagues, from the Gerentopsychiatry Center in Dusseldorf, Germany, gave twenty-nine patients suffering from anxiety 100 milligrams of kava extract [WS 1490] three times a day (Kinzler 1991). The study was done in a randomized, placebo-controlled, double-blind manner. The therapeutic efficacy was measured by the Hamilton Anxiety Scale and the Clinical Global Impression Scale. The results were noticeable within one week, and symptoms kept improving over the month of the study. No adverse reactions were caused by the kava during the four weeks of administration.

In 1996, another four-week double-blind, placebo-controlled study with forty-three females and fifteen males showed similar results (Lehmann 1996). In contrast to placebo, patients who received 70 milligrams of kavalactones three times a day were found to have a reduced amount of anxiety.

It would be interesting to do studies comparing the long-term therapeutic effects of kava with benzodiazepines or some of the newer antianxiety drugs such as buspirone.

5

THE KAVA EXPERIENCE

After treating patients with kava, talking to dozens of kava users, discussing its effects with doctors who recommend it to patients, and taking it myself off and on for a year, I have discovered that not everyone reacts exactly the same way to this herb. This is due to the fact that each of us has a different biochemistry. Furthermore, different products on the market may contain different amounts of constituents. The form of kava, whether liquid, tincture, or capsule, may also make a difference on how you feel, or how quickly you feel the effects. And finally, the dosage is important. Too low a dose won't produce an effect.

Most of the time, the effects of kava are noticed within an hour or two and can last several hours. A high dose can induce noticeable effects in a shorter period of time. If you are already relaxed and have no muscle tension, you won't notice the calming effects of kava as well as someone who is very tense and is already very anxious.

As a rule, the following are some common feelings that most users report:

- A state of relaxation, without reduction of mental acuity.
- Muscle relaxation.
- Feelings of peacefulness and contentment with mild euphoria.
- A few individuals on kava report a slight, temporary enhancement of visual acuity. Objects and people take on a sharper look. There's a mild improvement in awareness. I have personally noticed this on many occasions. Some users notice an enhancement of auditory acuity.
- Enhanced mental alertness and concentration.
- Most users notice being more sociable. Some report a slight opening of the heart, with an increased interest in getting to know other people and being close to them. A sense of harmony could be ex-

perienced with others at a party or meeting.

- Slightly more energy initially, followed by a need to slow down. Although sometimes temporary weakness or dizziness can be experienced.
- Some users report feeling sleepier. Whether you feel more alert or sleepy from kava ingestion depends on your individual biochemistry and also on the product you are using. Often there's a feeling of alertness and stimulation followed by being drowsy and sleepy hours later. Many people have the misconception that kava is a sedative. This herb actually causes alertness, at least initially. The sedation follows many hours later.

The fact that kava causes relaxation without sedation distinguishes it from many drugs used for anxiety (Xanax, Valium), since these drugs have a tendency to interfere with cognitive functioning. The lack of mental slowing allows kava to be used during the day. Albert, a forty-five-year-old stockbroker, tells me, "Whenever the trading becomes really hectic, I take a kava capsule containing 70 milligrams of kavalactones. Within forty-five minutes all signs of anxiety vanish, and a calm state of relaxation ensues for about two hours. Kava doesn't put me to sleep but just relaxes me while leaving my mind alert until the trading day is over."

Many individuals have a pleasant experience their very first time of using kava. Helen, a visitor from Vermont, says, "I was recently in California and was a dinner guest at a friend's house where I was served a very bitter, small-teacup amount of a beverage made from kava. After a while I experienced a very pleasant and relaxing sensation that seemed mildly narcotic. The evening went well, and at bedtime I quickly fell into a sound sleep. The next morning I felt amazingly refreshed (though still a bit buzzed) and had such a powerful dream during the night that I insisted on discussing it at the table."

On the other hand, I should note that some first-time users do not feel an effect from kava, or what they feel is minimal. Timothy, a twenty-five-year-old office manager, took a capsule containing 70 milligrams of kavalactones on three separate occasions without feeling any effects. He felt the kava only when he increased the dosage to three capsules. There are individuals who may need to take more than one pill to notice the effects of kava. However, once an effect is felt, often a lower dosage the next time can be more readily noticed.

If you are really interested in using kava, consult your physician and don't give up. Upon repeated use, you will find that the effects of the kava become more noticeable. Sometimes the effects are noticed only briefly, for a few minutes. A second dose taken at this time may be appropriate. Also, try different products if the first one or two do not give you the desired effect.

The highest amount I've personally taken is 500 milligrams of the kavalactones. I took this amount at 6 P.M. on the evening of my fortieth birthday. I then walked a mile with a friend to a restaurant near my home where I planned to meet several friends for dinner. I started noticing the alertness at about 7:30, followed by the urge to socialize. During the meal, I had two glasses of sake, the Japanese alcoholic drink made from fermented rice. After dinner, I walked back home and stayed up until midnight. To my surprise, instead of feeling sleepy, as I expected, I had a restless night. The following morning, I awoke early and felt surprisingly alert. This alertness lasted until noon. This convinced me that very high doses of kava could lead to alertness lasting more than twelve hours.

A very important point to keep in mind is that different products may produce different mental effects. If you are intent on using kava as a way to reduce anxiety, experiment with at least two or three different products. If you don't feel anything from one pill, you may find that two or three pills can provide the effect you're searching for.

Side effects are also possible and are discussed in a later chapter.

6

KAVA AND ANXIETY DISORDERS

As a rule, ingesting a kava pill or drinking the liquid preparation can induce a state of relaxation without loss of alertness. Inhabitants of the South Pacific used kava for ceremonial and recreational purposes. However, kava extracts can be used for therapeutic reasons. The study by Volz published in 1997 that I discussed in Chapter 4 has determined the effectiveness of kava on some forms of anxiety. Before I discuss the therapeutic uses of kava, it's important to define anxiety, the different ways it can manifest, and the different terminology used by doctors to define several subsets of this condition (Banazak 1997).

Anxiety is the term applied to a condition manifested by certain psychological and medical symptoms. The psychological state or symptoms include worry, hypervigilance, and occasional mild depression. Some of the physical symptoms are muscle tension, increased heart rate, and elevated blood pressure.

Stress and anxiety can be beneficial in terms of stimulating our brains and bodies to improve performance. However, excessive stress and anxiety can impair normal functioning. Both social and occupational performance can be affected.

The medical profession has categorized anxiety disorders in six ways.

ADJUSTMENT DISORDER WITH ANXIETY

This is the most common form of anxiety disorder. Almost everybody has had a stressful life event, such as death or severe illness in the family, divorce, financial difficulties, and so on. The immediate consequence of this stress is the onset of anxiety. As a rule, this type of anxiety is short-lived, often lasting no longer than a few months, and medicines are not needed to treat it. Counseling, having open talks with friends or family, and relaxation techniques are adequate to treat this condition. However, if the anxiety persists, is causing enduring problems with sleep, or is interfering with work performance, patients often visit their doctor for help. The medicines most often prescribed by doctors are the benzodiazepines, such as Xanax and Valium. These medicines do work; however, they have drawbacks. They are very sedating, interfere with mental clarity, and are potentially addictive. They may also interfere with memory.

Barbara, a forty-seven-year-old bookkeeper, went through a very difficult period during a divorce after a twenty-year marriage. "I couldn't function at work," she reported. "I kept staring at the ledger with all kinds of numbers, and all I could see was my husband's face. I tried a kava capsule containing 60 milligrams of kavalactones at the suggestion of a coworker, but it didn't help much. He recommended that I try two pills. The increase in dosage did make a difference. I used kava a few times a week for two months only on the days when I really felt I couldn't function without it. Sometimes I was so tense I needed three pills to relax me. I didn't want to go to a doctor and get a prescription drug. Thankfully, the kava was there when I needed help."

Kava is not always effective, though. Kevin, a forty-four-year-old vice president of an advertising company, is always tense and has been using Xanax off and on for many years.

"I gave kava a try along with other herbs supposed to help one relax. I found them lacking in real relief qualities. So, I'm back to my Xanax."

Kava does not work for everyone. However, there are a significant number of individuals with mild to moderate anxiety who will appreciate this herb's relaxing qualities.

GENERALIZED ANXIETY DISORDER

This condition is often chronic, lasting longer than a few months, and is associated with constant anxiety and worry. At least 4 percent of patients who visit doctors suffer from this condition. Most symptoms begin during one's teens or twenties, often as a consequence of a particular stress, and the symptoms persist for years. A genetic influence has not yet been clearly discovered. Perhaps the influence of an anxious mother or father, along with traumatic early life experiences, may be predisposing factors.

Most of the symptoms fluctuate up and down depending on the amount of stress the patient is under. Anxiety is often accompanied by mild to moderate depression and alcohol overuse.

Since generalized anxiety disorder lasts for

many years, an individual with a moderate to severe case may have to rely on medicines for a long time. There is the potential to become addicted to these medicines, with the accompanying medical and psychological problems associated with this addiction. If kava is found to be helpful in partially or mostly relieving the anxiety, then it could serve as a substitute for the stronger medicines such as barbiturates, benzodiazepines, or the newer antianxiety drugs such as buspirone (Buspar). The use of benzodiazepines and barbiturates leads to daytime sedation and interference with mental clarity. According to the 1998 *Physician's Desk Reference*, buspirone does not have a strong sedating property. However, it lacks muscle-relaxing abilities. Buspirone apparently works by influencing a specific type of serotonin receptor (5-HT1A) but has no apparent effect on benzodiazepine or GABA receptors.

Since the long-term use of each type of medicine could have harmful physiological effects, one option for someone who requires antianxiety medicines for many years is to take a particular medicine for a few months and then slowly switch to another. This way, the body is not exposed to the same type of drug, thus reducing the potential harm or damage to a particular organ. The possibility of developing addiction and tolerance is also reduced. If kava can be effectively used for a few weeks or months to reduce anxiety and thus obviate, at least temporarily, the need for pharmaceutical drugs, then we've done a great service to many patients. Michael W. Smith, M.D., of the Department of Psychiatry at Harbor-UCLA, in Los Angeles, agrees that this approach of switching from one medicine to another could potentially decrease the incidence of tolerance (personal communication).

The starting dose of kava in generalized anxiety disorders could be 70 milligrams of kavalactones twice a day. If needed, this can be gradually increased to 100 milligrams of kavalactones three times a day.

OBSESSIVE-COMPULSIVE DISORDER (OCD)

Do you know someone who washes his hands more often than necessary? A friend who keeps her house excessively clean? Someone who arranges his closet wardrobe very neatly? A spouse who thinks and talks about work all day and night? We certainly wouldn't consider any of these individuals to have a major problem. They may have type A personalities, we may occasionally call them obsessive or compulsive, but we don't categorize them as having a disorder.

However, when some of these traits are taken a step farther, and the compulsion and obsession go beyond what we consider normal in our society, it's time to call it a disorder. For instance, someone who washes his hands dozens of times a day, dusts the living room every hour, or keeps polishing the coffee table over and over has a problem. Physical symptoms could even develop. For instance, a person who repeatedly washes his hands could develop excessive dryness of the hands, itching, chafing, and even mild bleeding.

Obsessions are defined as recurrent and persistent thoughts, ideas, impulses, and images that are intrusive and senseless. Compulsions are repetitive and intentional behaviors that are performed in response to the obsessions. These obsessions and compulsions cause marked distress, are time-consuming, and interfere with the normal functioning of a person's day to day life.

The use of kava in OCD has not been formally evaluated, but it is worth a trial under the guidance of a health care practitioner.

PANIC DISORDER

Sudden episodes of overwhelming anxiety accompanied by a rapid heart rate can be extremely frightening. Over my many years of practicing medicine and working in emergency rooms, I have seen hundreds of relatively young individuals with panic disorders. A common account is that the person feels that he or she is having a heart attack or is going to die. It happened to my twenty-two-year-old cousin during her wedding ceremony. Suddenly she started breathing very hard and felt faint. Simply reassuring her that the panic attack would go away within a few minutes and that she wasn't going to die was enough to calm her down and return her to the altar.

If the panic disorder does not resolve quickly, an oral antianxiety agent such as Xanax or Valium is commonly prescribed. The use of kava has not been formally tested in panic disorders. It is unlikely that it would be effective in moderate or severe cases, but it might play a role in mild cases. Trudy, a twenty-five-year-old patient, tells me, "I have a mild case of panic disorder that leads me to hyperventilate whenever I'm about to go on an airplane. I've been planning this trip to Australia, and three weeks before the flight I started getting progressively nervous with temporary episodes of shallow breathing. I knew that if I didn't take a sedative, I would become progressively worse. So I started using kava, at a dose of 70 milligrams of the kavalactones, twice a day. It helped me relax and take my mind off the upcoming trip. The day of the trip I increased my dosage to 140 milligrams of the kavalactones and was able to survive the plane trip with very little apprehension."

Kava can certainly be tried before a particularly stressful event occurs, thus in some people preventing a possible panic attack. However, it doesn't work for everyone. Sarah, a twenty-two-year-old student, had a bad experience: "I was taking kava for irritable bowel syndrome and it was working well to relax my gut. However, I noticed that the frequency of my panic attacks increased. I think I'm just extremely sensitive, and the psychoactive properties of the kava made me a bit psychotic."

Certainly studies have to be done with kava and panic disorders before this herb can be universally recommended. We also have to appreciate the wide variety of human responses that can occur to the same medicine.

PHOBIAS

As a rule, phobias result from persistent fears that relatively harmless situations and objects can be injurious. Individuals can be afraid of animals (even harmless ones like frogs), heights, air travel, social encounters, and visits to a medical office. Phobias usually occur twice as commonly in women than men. Several common phobias are:

- agoraphobia—fear of being in a public place
- social phobia—fear of social embarrassment
- specific phobia—fear of a specific object or situation

One particular phobia that kava has the potential to benefit is social phobia. Kava has been traditionally known to enhance the urge to socialize. Therefore, a person who is withdrawn and shy would have a little help. Perhaps we'll find kava to be helpful in mild to moderate cases of social phobia.

The study that I discussed in Chapter 4 included patients who had been diagnosed with phobias (Volz 1997). Therefore, preliminary data appear to indicate that kava could play a role in helping certain individuals with phobias have an easier adjustment. Certainly more studies are needed before we can make any definitive recommendations.

POST-TRAUMATIC STRESS DISORDER

Many of us became aware of this diagnosis from the media attention paid to veterans of the Vietnam War. Some of these veterans had suffered enormous hardships, resulting in significant emotional and physical trauma. A few relive some of these traumas through recurrent nightmares. When these symptoms continue longer than a few weeks, a diagnosis of post-traumatic stress disorder (PTSD) is made. This condition can also result from other extremely stressful events outside the normal range of human experience, such as being a victim of a crime, sudden destruction of a home or community from a natural disaster, or seeing a person maimed or killed.

Kava has not been formally evaluated in the therapy of patients who suffer from PTSD. However, based on its ability to induce a peaceful relaxation, it could potentially be helpful.

MEDICAL CAUSES OF ANXIETY

There are several medical conditions that can induce symptoms similar to anxiety. Therefore, if you have persistent symptoms of anxiety and these symptoms are interfering with your day-to-day activities, you would benefit from a complete medical evaluation. The following are some common medical conditions that can mimic anxiety disorders.

- Angina: Chest pains due to mild heart attacks or spasm of the coronary arteries can sometimes be wrongly attributed to nervousness.
- Hyperthyroidism: Symptoms due to excessive thyroid hormone production include nervousness, irritability, difficulty concentrating, emotional lability, weight loss, sweating, and heart palpitations. A simple blood test can determine the levels of the thyroid hormones. A doctor would also check the size of the thyroid gland and look for other signs of hyperthyroidism such as bulging eyes and tremors.
- Hypoglycemia: Low blood sugar levels can induce the release of adrenaline-type

chemicals. Symptoms of hypoglycemia include nervousness, weakness, dizziness, and malaise.

- Pheochromocytoma: This is an uncommon medical disorder. A tumor in the adrenal glands leads to overproduction of epinephrine and norepinephrine, leading to rapid heart rate, sweating, headaches, and a rapid rise in blood pressure in response to minor stresses.

It's important to have a full medical evaluation to make sure there are no physical causes of anxiety before proceeding to any type of medication. A health care practitioner evaluating a patient with a suspected anxiety disorder would also need to inquire about caffeine, alcohol, and over-the-counter stimulant ingestion. Certain cold medicines contain stimulants such as pseudoephedrine. Even certain herbs can induce a state of nervousness, including mahuang, an herb that contains ephedra. High doses of St. John's wort can also induce nervousness. Amino acids, such as tyrosine and phenylalanine, increase energy and mood; however, nervousness, irritability, and heart palpitations are possible with higher dosages. DMAE (dimethylaminoethanol), a nutrient used for cognitive enhancement, can also cause anxiety and muscle tension in high dosages. High dosages of hormones such as pregnenolone and DHEA can induce irritability and anxiety in certain individuals.

Of course, before starting medicines, all other options to reduce anxiety should be attempted. These include counseling, cognitive-behavioral therapies, muscle relaxation techniques, relaxation books and tapes, guided imagery, yoga, breathing exercises, meditation, sincere talks with close friends and family, and vacations.

ANXIETY AND THE ELDERLY

At least 10 percent of older patients experience clinically important symptoms of anxiety (Hocking 1995). It is especially important in older individuals to rule out a medical problem causing the anxiety before proceeding to treat the psychological symptoms.

When deciding to recommend kava for seniors, physicians should at first start with a low dose such as 20 to 50 milligrams of kavalactones. The elderly are particularly susceptible to side effects to medicines, and over my many years of working in hospitals, I have come to realize that side effects to medicines are a lot more common than most people suspect. The metabolism in seniors is not as efficient as that of the young, and they are not able to break down and excrete many medicines in the proper time period. Thus, when given a normal dose of a benzodiazepine in the evening, some seniors are still extremely groggy in the morning, or can even exhibit various delusions or other psychotic symptoms.

7

KAVA OR VALIUM?

Over the past few decades, a number of pharmaceutical drugs have been introduced to the market in order to relieve stress and anxiety. Barbiturates, such as phenobarbital, were some of the first ones. They became very popular, but we soon learned the potential risks associated with their misuse. Barbiturates are prone to causing hangovers, tolerance, and dependence. Next came the benzodiazepine sedatives such as diazepam (Valium), chlordiazepoxide (Limbitrol), flurazepam (Dalmane), oxazepam (Serax), alprazolam (Xanax), lorazepam (Ativan), triazolam (Halcion), and others. These benzodiazepine medicines were safer than the barbiturates but still had a great risk for dependence and misuse. Fatalities frequently occurred by users of both barbiturates and benzodiazepines. We now have an additional antianxiety agent, buspirone (Buspar), which is not chemically related to the barbiturates or the benzodiazepines. Sometimes psychiatrists use certain antidepressants, such as tricyclics and serotonin reuptake inhibitors (such as Prozac) as antianxiety agents if there is depression associated with the anxiety.

With the growing popularity of kava, and with the publication of several articles in medical journals touting kava's positive results in combating anxiety, the question has been raised as to whether this herb can work as well as the pharmaceutical drugs. This is a very important medical issue because of the millions of individuals who have been prescribed drugs to treat their anxiety. If we find that kava can benefit these individuals, and subsequently they can go off their drugs to be placed on this herb, it would be a watershed event in medicine. This significance would mirror the effect St. John's wort has had in the therapy of depression, and what glucosamine has had in the therapy of osteoarthritis. A large number of older individuals have been able to reduce their reliance on nonsteroidal antiinflammatory drugs in favor of the safe and effective glucosamine.

KAVA VERSUS DRUGS

Even though both kava and diazepam (and other similar antianxiety benzodiazepinelike medicines) reduce muscle tension and are used to relieve anxiety, they have different effects on the brain and body.

In a study conducted in Hanover, Germany, twelve healthy volunteers were tested in a double-blind, crossover study to compare the effects of oxazepam (Serax) and an extract of kava root (Munte 1993). (Oxazepam is a benzodiazepine sedative similar to Valium.) Kava root extract was provided at 200 milligrams three times a day (kava extract WS 1490 was provided by Willmar Schwabe). The evaluation of the memory of the volunteers was done using a word recognition test. The subjects' task was to identify within a list of visually presented words those that were shown for the first time and those that were being repeated. The volunteers on oxazepam had a slowing of reaction time during the test of word recognition, while those on kava had a slight increase in the number of correct responses.

The following year, these same researchers repeated a study comparing kava to oxazepam

(Heinze, 1994). They again found that the administration of oxazepam decreased mental attention and the ability to process information while kava had a beneficial effect on mental clarity.

Advantages of Kava over Benzodiazepines

- Kava does not cause mental impairment or interfere with the ability to function at work or school. Memory stays intact.
- Kava has not been shown to be physically addictive. It can, however, be habit-forming in some users. Diazepam and its cousins have the potential to be both physically and psychologically addictive.
- No withdrawal symptoms have been associated with the abrupt cessation of kava use. Agitation and insomnia are common on withdrawal from benzodiazepines. Seizures and psychotic episodes can even occur.
- Death or severe illness from the exclusive use of kava has not been reported in the medical literature, whereas benzodiazepines cause central nervous system depression with the potential for respiratory and cardiac arrest on overdose.
- In cases where an antianxiety effect is

necessary without causing sedation, kava is the medicine of choice.

Disadvantages of Kava Compared to Benzodiazepines

- Kava is not as effective and consistent in inducing sleep and therefore cannot be considered a true hypnotic, meaning a sleep-inducing agent.
- In cases of anxiety associated with agitation, the drugs of choice are benzodiazepines. Kava is not as effective when a person is severely agitated and restless.
- Kava's effect on muscle relaxation is also not as powerful as that of diazepam. In cases of muscle sprains, such as severe neck or back sprain, kava does not work as well as diazepam.
- Kava is not as effective in patients who have severe anxiety.
- The effect from kava often lasts two to four hours, while many of the benzodiazepines can be effective for much longer period of time.
- The anticonvulsant effects of benzodiazepines are much more powerful.
- Kava is slower in action, and the effects generally take more than an hour or two

to start, whereas the effects from benzodiazepines are much quicker.

Many individuals who have tried both kava and pharmaceutical drugs have noticed the differences between the two. Daniel, a thirty-five-year-old patient who suffers from a mild case of post-traumatic stress disorder, says, "I found kava somewhat useful for combating the hypervigilance and rage of PTSD. My normal dose of kavalactones is 50 to 100 milligrams two to three times daily. The effect of kava is nowhere near as immediate and strong as your average benzodiazepine. After taking a kava dose, one does begin to feel more relaxed and a bit disconnected (another sign it's working is that sounds suddenly seem much louder; for some reason, it sharpens the hearing). It's nothing like Xanax and Valium, though. Normally it doesn't make one sleepy or goofy—instead you feel alert, but calm. I took kava for about three months and then found that I didn't need it anymore."

Dr. Hans-Peter Volz of the Department of Psychiatry at Jena University in Germany, is the author of the 1997 long-term study of kava use in anxiety disorders. He compares kava to tricyclic antidepressants (such as Elavil) and benzodiazepines (such as Valium): "As to benzodiazepines, their effectiveness in anxiety is beyond any doubt, and the short latency needed to establish the desired anxiolytic [relaxing] effect is a particular advantage. The two major drawbacks of this class of compounds are their dependency potential and their side-effect profile. Especially when administered on a long-term basis, benzodiazepines are difficult to withdraw. In this regard, kava is non-problematic. Withdrawal symptoms or dependency developments are not known. Also, in our trial, no withdrawal symptoms occurred in the last trial phase.

"Tricyclic antidepressants [such as Elavil], also widely used to treat anxiety disorders, have major side-effects, especially for higher doses, which account for a decreased compliance, and direct cardiotoxic effects which make it impossible to administer them to patients suffering from severe cardiac conduction disturbances. Such side effects are not known with respect to kava."

What about driving a car? Dr. Volz continues, "The side-effect profile of benzodiazepines, with drowsiness as the predominant symptom, leads to restrictions in driving vehicles or operating machinery. For kava-kava, the results show no detrimental influence of this compound on various psychometric parameters." However, it is important to note that studies have not been published giving kava to drivers and then checking their actual performance. If you're a first-time user, do not drive a car after taking kava. Your first time should be done when you are home.

Considering the factors mentioned above, it may be wise to consider the use of kava as first-line therapy in certain anxiety disorders. If you are currently on a tranquilizer, please remember that anytime you try to change from a prescription medicine to an herbal product, it is best to do so under the guidance of a health care professional.

8

THE LESS-STRESS, FEEL-GOOD HERB FOR EVERYDAY TENSION

There are many situations likely to make us stressed out and anxious. The use of kava could potentially reduce the anxiety associated with these stressful events, thus minimizing any worry and unpleasantness. For instance, David Essel, the host of the nationally syndicated show *David Essel Live*, says, "While I was writing a book proposal, I felt very stressed. There were deadlines to meet. Taking kava daily for a period of seven days took the edge off and I was able to be more productive."

Without a doubt, stress can profoundly influence the rate at which our brain cells age and become damaged. The area of the brain called the hippocampus is involved in memory storage. This area actually shrinks when the brain is exposed to too high a dose of stress hormones. Stress affects not only our brain cells but also the rest of the cells of our body. Mind you, a little stress is healthy because it challenges our brain and body to perform better. However, if it becomes excessive, there comes a point when our organs become exhausted and breakdowns can occur.

Stress is known to alter the amount and type of steroid hormones produced. This can lead to a failure in the maintenance of ideal hormonal balances. For example, an excess of cortisol can have significant negative consequences, including increases in blood sugar levels. This additional sugar is acquired by cortisol's inhibition of protein synthesis in muscles. Excess cortisol also inhibits the immune system and causes calcium loss, leading to osteoporosis.

In fact, excess cortisol, by crippling the immune system, increases the rate of infections. Processes that repair tissues can be shut down; sleep is interfered with; bones can become osteoporotic; and there could even be an increase in cancer risk. Certain cancers, cervical cancer for example, are partly caused by the human papilloma virus. Since stress interferes with the immune system, virus-causing cancers could get a foothold and start growing at a rapid rate.

Even though, as a rule, most of us are not involved in demanding physical labor, we are exposed to an enormous amount of psychological stress: We drive to work in the morning in horn-honking heavy traffic. Our work involves difficult bosses, deadlines, phone calls to return, and projects to complete. We have the traffic again on the way back home, dinner to prepare, active children to keep under control, feed, and nurture, bills to pay, and a home and garden to maintain. Sometimes there are social conflicts: disputes with relatives, friends, and loved ones. To add further insult, most people don't get enough hours of restful sleep and are therefore still stunned in the morning when the alarm clock blares the onset of another hectic day. It's enough to make our adrenal glands cry "uncle!"

Kava, if used appropriately, could help us reduce the stress in our lives, and it can even be used to prevent or decrease the amount of stress or anxiety we anticipate being exposed to.

BOARDING A PLANE

For a short flight, a one-time kava dose two to three hours before boarding should be enough.

For a longer flight, you may need a second dose during the flight. There are individuals who start getting nervous days before an upcoming trip. The use of kava for a few days prior to the trip could be helpful in reducing this worry.

If the flight is overnight, and you want to sleep on the plane, then kava could be counterproductive if it causes you to be alert. In these situations, melatonin can work well, since it will help you sleep and also readjust your sleep cycle. You could also take a small amount of kava (70 milligrams or less of the kavalactones) a couple of hours before boarding, then take the melatonin about a half hour to an hour before you plan to sleep. The melatonin would work well in the sublingual form, at a dose of 0.5 milligram up to 5 milligrams. The small amount of kava should not interfere with sleep.

Valerian (see Chapter 15) is another sedative herb to consider for use during flights.

A JOB INTERVIEW

Kava can be taken about two to three hours before the interview, unless the job specifications require a person to act "hyper."

THE DENTIST'S CHAIR

Kava is an ideal supplement to take before going to the dentist. Not only does it help you relax but it also acts as a mild analgesic. Kava paste applied topically could even be used after certain types of dental work to numb the teeth or gums. Ask your dentist first whether there are any contraindications to use kava paste for your particular condition.

Benzodiazepines also work well for this situation; however, the excessive sedation may interfere with driving to and from the dentist's office.

GOING ON A DATE

Mumbling and sweating rarely impress your date. Then there's the first-time visit to meet the potential future in-laws. Kava could come to the rescue.

ATTENDING A PARTY

If you're shy when meeting new people, raise a hearty toast to kava. John, a forty-year-old Webmaster, says, "I've drunk kava in the evening during get-togethers with friends. Kava makes me feel very mellow, comfortable, and sociable. It's easy to engage in conversations. Barriers go down and there's a feeling of connection to people. I feel more open, attuned, and aware. If I drink too much, the next day I notice having a slight headache."

It would be interesting to observe over the next few years whether kava will partially substitute for alcohol at social gatherings. One advantage that kava has over alcohol is that it does not induce aggression. Fights and conflicts are extremely rare in kava bars on the Pacific islands compared to bars that serve alcohol.

GIVING A SPEECH

Since kava can help you relax without affecting mental clarity, it is a good option to take before giving a speech. Propranolol (Inderal), available by prescription only, is another medicine that works very well. Twenty to forty milligrams of propranolol before a speech or television appearance can be tremendously helpful in preventing rapid heart rate and sweating.

BEFORE MEETINGS OR BEFORE COUNSELING SESSIONS

Linda Ligon, the president of Interweave Press in Loveland, Colorado, says, "Kava provides a leveling of mood. We sometimes use it at the office before meetings. It makes us kinder and gentler. It provides a subtle, uplifting effect, sometimes with a mild euphoria."

Kava has been used for centuries in the Pacific islands as a drink provided to chiefs before and during their meetings with other leaders. Terry Willard, Ph.D., president of Wild Rose College of Natural Healing in Calgary, Canada, reports, "Our counseling department gives kava an hour before a session to couples who are having marital difficulties. As a consequence, there are fewer arguments between them. It's a great arbitration herb."

Couples could even decide to set time out once a week, or once a month, to take kava and then have a frank discussion to go over any unresolved issues that had come up during this period.

Over time you can discover other situations that are particularly stressful for you, and you can experiment to see if kava is of benefit. There are certain situations where being a little nervous can be helpful, since it gives us an adrenaline rush to perform better. For instance, taking kava before an audition for a theater or acting role could be counterproductive if the role requires boisterous and energetic acting.

There are certain jobs that are inherently stressful. It's quite possible the occasional use of kava could provide some relief. For instance, accountants could find kava helpful during tax season, lawyers may appreciate this herb during prolonged and exhausting legal battles, while stockbrokers could use kava to wind down after a particularly stressful day on Wall Street.

9

KAVA FOR MILD DEPRESSION

Even though kava has been studied mostly as an antianxiety agent, it does have mood-elevating properties. Users notice a mild euphoria or a sense of well-being. Therefore, the use of kava could be considered in cases of mild depression. Since kava has relaxing properties, it could be particularly helpful when the depression is associated with anxiety or nervousness. Therefore, if you have a mild case of depression, kava might be an appropriate herb for you to use temporarily, such as for a few weeks. However, you might also consider the use of the herb St. John's wort, which has been more thoroughly evaluated in the therapy of depression.

One disadvantage of kava as an antidepressant is that its effects last only a few hours. Generally, most medicines used to treat depression should have an effect that lasts most of the day, or even overnight. For instance, if you take a St. John's wort pill in the morning, you can often feel the mood-elevating or energy-producing effect of this herb late into the evening. Another disadvantage of kava is that, after a few hours of alertness and mood elevation, it can, in some individuals, induce sleepiness and lethargy. This property may be beneficial if kava is taken in the late afternoon or early evening. However, if the kava is taken during the day, a person with depression may feel overly tired and lethargic in the afternoon, unless a second dose of kava is taken at that time.

You may find products in vitamin stores that include both kava and St. John's wort. Since no research has been published with this combination, it is difficult to predict what effects they will have. However, since it is unlikely that any formal research will be done using these herbs together, our primary source of information in the near future will be from anecdotes. You may want to try this combination under the guidance of a health care practitioner familiar with herbal therapy.

Before you try combining herbs, though, it

is preferable that you experiment with kava alone. Learn as much as you can about the different effects of this herb on your body and mind. Take the herb at different times of the day and in different dosages. Try at least a couple of different products since there may be differences in their effects. Also try at least two different forms of a product before you form a definitive opinion on its benefits. For instance, take kava capsules, and if you don't find them effective, try the tincture form.

Once you are familiar with one herb, let's say kava, go off it and learn about another one, such as St. John's wort. Take St. John's wort in the morning at a dose of 300 milligram of the 0.3 percent (hypericin content) standardized extract. Take this dosage of St. John's wort each morning for one week. If your mood is still lower than you hoped for, you can take a second pill of St. John's wort midday. Once you are familiar with the effects of St. John's wort, you can then consider adding kava. As mentioned previously, kava could be particularly helpful if your depression is associated with anxiety or nervousness. But there's another reason why kava could be advantageous when combined with St. John's wort. In some people, St. John's wort can lead to irritability, restlessness, or even mild anxiety. If high doses give you these symptoms, you can take a lower dose and combine it with kava. This way, instead of relying exclusively on St. John's wort, you take advantage of the properties of both herbs. Genny, a thirty-year-old accountant from Los Angeles, says, "I've taken various prescribed antidepressants, Prozac, Zoloft, and the like, but did not find them particularly effective . . . and I really disliked the side effects. I've started taking St. John's wort with kava root in it and have been feeling much better. Apparently, the kava works rather quickly—within a couple of days—whereas the St. John's wort takes about four weeks to build up in the system and take full effect." Michael W. Smith, M.D., of the Department of Psychiatry at Harbor-UCLA, in Los Angeles, believes that since kava and St. John's wort influence a different set of brain chemicals, there are theoretically no known neurochemical contraindications to the combined use of these two herbs (personal communication). Kenneth Boch, M.D., a physician who practices complimentary medicine in Rhinebeck, New York, reports that in his limited experience, kava does help take the edge off the occasional irritability or anxiety consequent to the use of St. John's wort.

The whole process of combining herbs is

not yet a science. It may require a great deal of experimentation. Many people enjoy this process. Most of us like to have a sense of control over our body. We often like the attempt to be our own doctor instead of constantly relying on time-consuming and expensive office visits. There's no reason to burden the already bursting-at-the-seams medical system by constantly making appointments with doctors for minor conditions. By learning how to treat minor illnesses ourselves through natural methods and supplements, we can relieve the pressure on doctors and hospitals and reduce the overall cost of medical care. Medical insurance rates could also come down. However, self-experimentation is not a good option in cases of moderate or severe depression. A doctor's supervision is crucial during these times.

In addition to St. John's wort, there are other natural supplements touted to improve mood, and they should certainly be considered in combination therapy with kava. I recommend that you take a B complex vitamin supplement somewhere between one to five times the RDA (recommended daily allowance). The use of B vitamins has been shown to improve mood (Benton 1995). If you are in your late forties or older, going on hormone replacement therapy with pregnenolone or DHEA could offer mood-elevating benefits (see *Pregenolone: Nature's Feel Good Hormone* for details). However, hormones should be used only in very low dosages and only under the guidance of a health care practitioner.

The use of kava with pharmaceutical antidepressant medicines such as Prozac, Paxil, and Zoloft has not been evaluated. In some cases, these medicines can cause restlessness or slight anxiety. It would be interesting to explore the use of kava with a lower dosage of these medicines. This way, kava could help induce relaxation yet still offer some mood elevation.

Several other supplements have mild mood-elevating properties. These include the herbs ginkgo and ginseng, the nutrients phosphotidylserine and 5-hydroxytryptophan, the amino acids tyrosine and phenylalanine, and the antioxidant lipoic acid. Of course, let's not neglect exercise as a powerful way to enhance mood.

One additional pharmaceutical medicine that has the potential to positively influence mood is selegiline. It is known by the product name Eldepryl, and the research name deprenyl. Selegiline is thought to improve mood through its actions on the dopaminergic system. It is often used in the therapy of patients who have Parkinson's disease. The combination of kava and selegiline has not been tested.

Each nutrient, herb, drug, and hormone has advantages and disadvantages. I think that for too long Western medicine has mostly relied on monotherapy (the exclusive use of one drug or medicine) in the therapy of depression. Doctors practicing Oriental medicine have often used several herbs in combination while treating a particular condition. The disadvantage to the use of monotherapy is that when higher and higher dosages of a medicine are required to treat the depression, the possibility of side effects increases proportionally. By appropriately using low dosages of more than one medicine or supplement, one can theoretically reap similar, or better, benefits while minimizing the risks. For instance, one benefit of pregnenolone is that it enhances visual and auditory perception. When combined with the mood-elevating properties of St. John's wort, a dramatic antidepressant effect and sense of well-being could be realized, along with an enhanced sense of visual appreciation. However, high doses of both pregnenolone and St. John's wort can, in some people, lead to restlessness and anxiety. Kava could take the edge off this side effect. DHEA has the advantage of improving sex drive, while St. John's wort has minimal influence on libido. Also, by using low doses of DHEA and preg- nenolone, the likelihood of a side effect, such as acne, is minimized. As you can see, one can tailor the combination of these nutrients and hormones to suit the individual patient. It may take trial and error to find the ideal combina- tion. The challenge becomes in finding a health care practitioner who is willing to guide you while you are experimenting with these com- binations.

Note that the use of combinations of sup- plements to treat depression is very new and there's a lot medicine has yet to learn about this approach. Caution advises us to proceed at a slow rate in adding and combining sup- plements, and the dosages used initially should be very small. The guidance of a health care practitioner is strongly advised.

10
KAVA AND INSOMNIA

Even though certain individuals find a small dose of kava helpful as a sleep aid, the sedating and hypnotic (sleep-inducing) effects of kava are not universally consistent. There are variations in individual responses to the herb's sedating effects. Most users feel very alert and report that the ingestion of kava actually interferes with their sleep. The most commonly reported effect is that kava initially makes one more alert, but after a few hours there's a change to being more sedated. Don't take kava right before bed and expect it immediately to make you sleepy as does a pharmaceutical sleeping pill or melatonin. Early evening dosing would be a good option. The dosage could also make a difference. A lower dose in certain individuals could be mildly relaxing and help with sleep onset, while a higher dose could well lead to feeling wide awake. Also keep in mind that there are several varieties of kava plants and countless numbers of kava products. Some could be more sedating than others.

Kava is not known to cause hangovers. David Snow, the host of the radio show *Doctor Health* in Honolulu, says, "The effects are subtle but I often sleep better with kava. I feel super when I wake up in the morning without the residual grogginess."

Kava can be combined with several supplements, melatonin, and herbs. As a rule, keep the kava dose to less than 70 milligrams of kavalactones in the late evening if you want to avoid insomnia. If you happen to have taken a high dose of kava in late evening, and you are still alert by bedtime, melatonin can be a wonderful savior. Melatonin, in a dosage of 0.3 to 1 milligram is best taken about half an hour to an hour before bed. You can take the regular pills, the sublingual tablets that melt in the mouth, the liquid time-release pills, or even the tea form.

Valerian is another option to use at night if the kava is keeping you alert. If you happen to be very alert, it is unlikely that some of the milder-acting sedative herbs such as chamomile and passionflower will be adequate to counteract the effects.

Another supplement available over the counter is 5-hydroxytryptophan (5-HTP), which is a precursor to the important mood chemical in the brain known as serotonin. 5-HTP has antidepressant abilities, although more studies need to be done to confirm the preliminary findings. 5-HTP is sedating and sleep promoting; therefore, taking between 10 and 50 milligrams a half hour to an hour before bed can induce a calm sleep. Many users notice that they yawn within a half hour of taking 5-HTP. (See *5-HTP: Nature's Serotonin Solution* for details.)

Please remember that any time you combine two substances that have a sedative effect, the initial dosages used should be minimal until you learn how these supplements influence your particular chemistry. Each person has a unique response.

Jet lag is another condition for which kava has anecdotally been touted to be helpful, although it wouldn't address the primary problem of readjusting the circadian clock as well as would melatonin, or perhaps 5-HTP.

One should not regularly rely on the use of pills to induce sleep. Here are a few simple steps to more restful nights.

TEN TIPS TO FORTY WINKS

1. Expose yourself to morning light by taking a walk. This tends to shorten the sleep cycle so that when you go to bed at night it is easier to fall asleep.
2. Exercise has the tendency to shorten the sleep cycle. The best times to work out are in the late afternoon or early evening. Exercise may delay sleep if performed within three or so hours before bedtime.
3. When body temperature is raised in the late evening, it falls at bedtime, facilitating sleep. A sauna or hot bath for at least ten minutes an hour or two before bed serves this purpose.
4. Taking daily naps longer than one hour or after 4 P.M. makes you less sleepy at bedtime.
5. Caffeine in any form (sodas, chocolate, coffee, or certain teas) is best avoided after dinner.
6. Consumption of alcohol in the evening may help one fall asleep, but the sleep is often fragmented and light.
7. Eating a small or moderate late-night

snack within two hours before bedtime may actually promote sleep, especially if the meal includes carbohydrates (such as whole grains, legumes, fruits, pasta, or rice).

8. Strenuous mental activity should stop at least one hour before bed and the mind allowed to switch to easy reading or watching a comedy film or TV show.

9. Use earplugs to muffle noises.

10. Try one or more relaxation techniques. When you are in bed lying on your back, shake and loosen a leg and foot. Take a few slow deep breaths by expanding your belly. Shake and loosen the other leg and foot and then return to your abdomen for a few more relaxed breaths. Proceed with this relaxation to your arms, shoulders, and neck. Now relax your facial muscles, especially the muscles around the eyes and mouth. Remember to return to your breath after relaxing each muscle group. Before you know it you'll be drifting into your adventure-filled unconscious.

There are times when, in spite of our very best attempts, we do not feel sleepy at bedtime. Instead of tossing and turning all night, the use of natural herbs and supplements can help us enormously in getting the restful sleep that our body needs. I also do not have objections to using a pharmaceutical sleep medicine. In my opinion, it is healthier occasionally to take a sleeping pill and have a deep, restful sleep and feel energized the next day than spend a long night alert in the dark hoping for daylight to come.

One interesting effect of kava that has anecdotally been reported is that some users notice slightly enhanced dreams. Melatonin is definitely known to produce vivid dreaming. The influence of the combination of melatonin and kava on dreams is currently not known.

11

CLINICAL USES OF KAVA

The antianxiety effects of kava have been well researched, but compounds in this herb may have several other therapeutic properties. Unfortunately, the medical uses of kava in disorders not directly related to anxiety have not been thoroughly evaluated, but we have a few studies that give us hints regarding other conditions in which kava could play a medicinal role.

AS A PAINKILLER

A study in mice has shown kava to have mild pain-reducing properties (Jamieson 1990). A number of extracts from kava were found to be effective, including kawain, dihydrokawain, methysticin, and dihydromethysticin. How these extracts work is not fully known, but they do not appear to involve the same brain chemical system as regular painkillers like codeine or morphine.

When I worked in the emergency room, I treated quite a few people who were suffering from narcotic overdose. The proper treatment, in addition to inducing vomiting to get the pills out, is to give an intravenous injection of naloxone. When this medicine is injected, it goes to many parts of the body, including the lungs and heart, and reverses the effects of narcotics or opiates.

In the mouse study mentioned above, the injection of naloxone was not effective in reversing the painkilling activities of kava extracts. The researchers state, "The analgesia induced by kava occurs via non-opiate pathways."

There are many people who are allergic to painkillers such as codeine. Perhaps we will find that kava is useful in mild painful conditions for these individuals. We may also find that kava can be used in combination with aspirin, acetaminophen, and lower dosages of narcotic painkillers for a synergistic effect. Certainly more research is needed.

Specific conditions that some patients have

used kava include headaches, neck pain, back pain, temperomandibular joint syndrome (TMJ), toothaches, and menstrual cramps. In most cases, users should not expect significant relief as they would from a codeine pill. However, kava could provide enough of a relief to make the discomfort tolerable.

Another way that kava could be used is as a topical anesthetic. Kava can numb nerves of mucous membranes. This property could be taken advantage of in terms of using kava as a topical anesthetic in cases of toothaches or gum pain.

MENOPAUSAL SYMPTOMS

Menopause causes a variety of hormonal changes that can disturb mood and cause tenseness. Estrogen can be helpful during this period, and so can certain natural compounds.

At the 1996 American Heart Association's annual scientific conference, researchers discussed the growing evidence that soybean ingestion may relieve some of the symptoms of menopause. Dr. Gregory Burke, of Bowman Gray School of Medicine in Winston-Salem, North Carolina, reported that women suffering hot flashes had less intense symptoms after ingesting soy protein.

Forty-three women age forty-five to fifty-five, who suffered daily bouts of hot flashes or night sweats were given 20 grams of powdered soy protein for six weeks. Then they were given 20 grams of powdered carbohydrate for six weeks. The volunteers were not aware until after the study whether they had consumed soy protein or carbohydrate.

Although the frequency of hot flashes was not reduced, the severity of the episodes was. The researchers believe that the key ingredient of soy protein is phytoestrogen, the plant form of human estrogen. Soy estrogens act on the same chemical targets or receptors in the body as human estrogens, although they are less potent.

Does kava play a role in easing menopausal symptoms? In a double-blind, placebo-controlled study involving twenty women with menopause-related symptoms, kava extract (WS 1490, containing 100 milligrams of kava) was given three times per day (Warnecke 1991). Several psychological tests were done throughout the study to monitor mood and anxiety. The participants were also asked to keep diaries. The study lasted eight weeks, but there were already significant benefits noted within the first week. Most of the women reported improved mood and well-being, and less anxiety. The researcher states, "The course of such further parameters as depressive mood, subjective well-being, severity of the disease, and the climacteric symptomatology throughout the period of treatment demonstrate a high level of efficacy of kava extract WS 1490 in neurovegetative and psychosomatic dysfunctions in the climacteric, associated with very good tolerance of the preparation."

It would be interesting to do a study combining both soy products and kava to find out if, by using natural supplements, women during their climacteric could reduce their dosage of estrogen.

PREMENSTRUAL SYNDROME (PMS)

PMS occurs, to some degree, in one-third of women of childbearing age. Symptoms include irritability, increased aggressiveness, cravings for sweet or salty foods, nervousness, mood swings, difficulty in concentrating, fatigue, tenderness of the breasts, and abdominal bloating.

These symptoms appear during the latter half of the menstrual cycle and disappear with the onset of menstruation. The exact causes of PMS are not fully known, but hormonal imbalances or "abnormal" responses to the fluctuating hormonal levels (such as progesterone) during the late part of the menstrual cycle are thought to be involved.

The role of kava in PMS has not been formally evaluated. Anecdotal reports indicate that some users notice partial relief of some aspects of anxiety and irritability associated with the syndrome.

URINARY TRACT INFECTIONS

One of the most annoying aspects of urinary tract infections is the burning sensation in the urethra. Kava, acting as an anesthetic, is thought to decrease this discomfort. However, kava does not address the actual infection. Studies have indicated that bacteria can grow in cultures despite the presence of kavalactones (Hansel 1968).

Lise Alschuler, N.D., Chair of the Botanical Medicine Department at Bastyr University in Seattle, Washington, says, "An interesting use of kava is as an analgesic (pain medicine) for bladder infections. It has a numbing effect to the bladder mucosa. I prescribe a lower dose four or five times a day. This is, of course, in addition to other medicines that fight the bladder infection."

ANTISEIZURE

In laboratory studies, extracts of kava have been shown to suppress the release of the brain chemical glutamate and thus reduce the tendency of brain cells to get excited (Gleitz 1996). This means that kava extracts may theoretically reduce the incidence of seizures. However, we won't know the clinical significance of this laboratory finding on isolated brain cells until actual human studies are done. It's unlikely that kava alone would be adequate therapy for convulsions. However, this study does indicate that there is currently no contraindication for a patient who has a tendency for seizures to take kava.

The appropriateness of kava use in individuals who are currently on antiseizure medicines is not known. Several medicines are prescribed for seizure disorders, including phenytoin, phenobarbital, valproic acid, diazepam, clonazepam, and carbamazepine. The interaction of kava with these medicines has not been evaluated. Could the use of kava reduce the dosages required for these medicines? It is hoped that future research will examine kava's role in the therapy of epilepsy.

AS A BLOOD THINNER

Dr. J. Gleitz and colleagues, from the Institute for Natural Studies at the University of Ulm, in Germany, have discovered that a chemical in the kava root, specifically kavain, has blood-thinning abilities.

One of the fatty acids found in blood, called arachidonic acid (AA), has the ability to induce platelets to stick together. An excess amount of AA can lead to a blood clot forming in the cardiovascular system. In a laboratory test tube, Dr. Gleitz added arachidonic acid to platelets and found them to clump very easily. However, when these same platelets were exposed to kavain, one of the components in the kava plant, five minutes before the addition of AA, no such clumping of platelets occurred (Gleitz 1997). The clinical significance of this property is currently not known, nor do we know how strong the anticlotting properties of kava extracts are compared to aspirin.

Another herb known to have anticlotting abilities is ginkgo biloba, often used to improve memory. You should let your health care practitioner be aware of all the supplements you are taking in case there are some interactions.

AS AN ANTIINFLAMMATORY AGENT

Another property of kava identified by Dr. Gleitz is its ability to prevent the formation of prostaglandin E2 and thromboxane A2, by respectively inhibiting the action of the enzymes cyclooxygenase and thromboxane synthase. Practically speaking, the blocking of these enzymes would lead to a decrease in inflammation. Certain nonsteroidal antiinflammatory drugs are known to be effective in blocking the action of these enzymes. Traditionally, Pacific islanders have used kava to decrease symptoms of diseases associated with inflammation, such as rheumatism. Certainly more research is necessary before we can recommend the use of kava in noninfectious inflammatory disorders.

FIBROMYALGIA AND MUSCLE ACHES

Also known as fibrositis, fibromyalgia is characterized by various aches and pains in muscles, subcutaneous tissues, ligaments, and tendon insertions. Certain parts of the body have tender points. Joints are not involved. No currently known cause or associated disorder has been determined. The diagnosis is made clinically since no blood studies or laboratory tests can pinpoint the disorder.

Studies evaluating the therapeutic potential of kava in fibromyalgia have not been published. However, a few people who have this disorder have reported mild relief in their symptoms from this herb. This is only anecdotal evidence, and we certainly need more data to confirm these findings.

The same is true of muscle spasms. Some individuals have found kava to be helpful. Here's the account of Jerry, a sixty-year-old patient: "I have arthritis and associated muscle spasms. I was quite amazed at how kava was helpful for the muscle spasms. The effects lasted for several hours. It had such a noticeable effect, with minimal side effects."

GASTROINTESTINAL DISORDERS

Kavain, one of the kavalactones in the kava plant, has been found in the laboratory to induce relaxation of isolated guinea pig ileum smooth muscle cells (Seitz 1997). (The ileum, along with the duodenum and the jejunum, is part of the small intestine.) There are a number of anxiety disorders that produce gastrointestinal symptoms due to overactivity of the intestinal smooth muscle cells; one is irritable bowel syndrome (IBS). Traditionally, Pacific islanders have used kava for certain intestinal conditions. Kava has not been formally tested in IBS, but there appears to be a biochemical basis that kava offers some benefits in inducing relaxation of the intestines in anxiety-induced or aggravated gastrointestinal disorders.

IN CHILDREN

The use of kava in children has not been studied. In cases of mild sleep disorders in infants, chamomile is a good option (see Chapter 18). For slightly older children, an occasional small dose of valerian (see Chapter 15) could be helpful if the child really needs a sleep aid on a particular evening. The response of a child to kava cannot be easily predicted. Therefore, for the time being it is best to try alternatives before resorting to kava.

However, there are anecdotal reports that the occasional use of kava could be helpful. Danielle, the mother of an autistic child, says, "Sammy was a terrible sleeper until we tried melatonin. I had read about it at the Center for the Study of Autism Web site. It worked great until he started to build a tolerance to it. We stopped the melatonin for a period of two weeks. I was starting to get worried because Sammy was having insomnia again. The lady at the health food store recommended I try liquid kava. I had tried the valerian, but it did not work well. The kava worked really well. I give it to him about two hours before bed and again right before bedtime. The first dose calms him down, so he doesn't get pumped up before bedtime. The second sends him right off. I am now considering a combination of kava and melatonin, using a portion of the recommended dose just to see what happens."

It is best to avoid using any sleeping aid regularly due to the potential of developing tolerance.

Kava could theoretically also be helpful in children when used occasionally for a particular stressful occasion such as the first day at a new school or visiting a family member who's in the hospital. However, you should consult your family health care practitioner before trying kava with children.

12

THE RIGHT DOSE

The amount of kava to take depends on your purpose for using this herb and your individual sensitivity to the effects of kavalactones. Here are some guidelines to help you get started.

Whenever a new medicine, herb, or supplement is first tried, it is always best to start with low dosages and build up. This cautious approach should minimize any untoward reactions. You may be particularly sensitive to the psychoactive effects of the supplement, or be on a medicine that interacts with it, or even have an allergy to the compounds in the pill. Here's a step-by-step guide to follow.

1. Start with a one-time dose between 40

and 70 milligrams of kavalactones. For instance, if your bottle says it contains 150 milligrams of kava with a content of kavalactones at 30 percent, then 150 milligrams times 30 percent equals about 45 milligrams. Taking your first kava dose in the late afternoon or evening is a good option. It is best to take it on a day when you are home and don't need to drive or operate heavy machinery.

2. If this low dose provides no effects within two to three hours, then you can take an additional capsule.

3. The next day, if you did not notice an effect from the kava, you can take more. If you took 50 milligrams of the kavalactones, you can increase your dose to 70 to 80 milligrams. Again, if there's been no effect in two or three hours, you can take another capsule.

4. If kava did not provide you with any effects the first couple of days, then you could increase your dosage to 100 milligrams of kavalactones. You should notice effects at this dosage, although there are individuals who require higher amounts initially to feel something. Once you feel an effect, you can gener-

ally be more attuned and feel similar effects on lower dosages. In cases of severe anxiety, some people may respond only to very high doses, such as 150 to 200 milligrams of kavalactones two or three times a day.

WHAT YOU WILL FIND IN YOUR VITAMIN OR RETAIL STORE

It can be a daunting experience going to a large health food store with aisles and aisles and shelves and shelves, full of thousands of supplements from dozens of different companies. If you are new to the field of vitamins, minerals, herbs, and supplements, you are likely to be overwhelmed. Fortunately, most stores have a manager or owner who can guide you in selecting the product that suits you best. However, some stores don't provide anyone who can help you make the proper selection. In the long run, it is preferable if you learn the details about how many supplements are available and the best forms to take.

Many herbs, including kava, are available in stores in a number of forms; including pills, capsules, liquid, tincture, powder, root, and tea. The ideal form of taking an herb depends whether the active compounds in the herb are fat- or water-soluble. If they are water-soluble, drinking the tea is adequate. If the active compounds are fat-soluble, then a laboratory needs to have a process that can extract these fat-soluble compounds. In the case of kava, the capsules sold over the counter do include the fat-soluble kavalactones. Tinctures are made by soaking the root material in an alcoholic liquor such as brandy or gin, which also has the ability to dissolve the kavalactones.

As a rule, the content of kavalactones in the kava root can vary from 3 to 20 percent. Thus, many manufacturers take extracts of the root to provide a standard percentage of kavalactones in their product. Often, the percentage of kavalactones in these extracts is about 30 percent. If a container lists, for example, 150 milligrams kava root extract of 30 percent kavalactones, you can compute that it yields about 45 milligrams of kavalactones. But when the percentage of the kavalactones is not listed, it's hard to tell how much of the active ingredients you are getting. Keep in mind that each product has a different amount of kavalactones and other active ingredients depending on how the root is processed and how the active ingredients are extracted. Some companies add extracts of stems and leaves, which alters the kavalactone content. However, more important than knowing the exact amount of the kavalactones your are ingesting is determining how you are reacting to a particular product. After experimenting with several products, you can choose the one that best works for you.

COMBINATIONS

Kava can be found in a number of products, combined with a variety of other relaxing herbs. Some of the common herbs mixed with kava are valerian, passionflower, chamomile, and St. John's wort.

TINCTURES

Many of the active ingredients in kava are soluble in alcohol. Therefore, one way of extracting these ingredients is by soaking the powdered or chopped root in an alcoholic liquor such as brandy or gin. The purpose of the alcohol is to dissolve the active ingredients from the herb into the solution. The proportion of alcohol used, and the type of alcohol, can vary among manufacturers. One particular company reports this on the bottle: "Content: Made from freshly harvested kava kava root, pure grain alcohol (60 to 70% alcoholic content) and distilled spring water. Harvested from the island of Vanuatu, where the finest kava in the world grows. Suggested use: Take 15–20 drops of extract in a small amount of warm water 3 times daily as needed."

Tinctures may be a good way of taking kava, but it's difficult to know how much of the active ingredients you are ingesting. They usually come in a dropper bottle containing one fluid ounce. For a quick effect you can place a dropperful under your tongue. Expect some facial grimaces, since the taste can be biting, numbing, burning, and terrible—all at the same time. Torrey, a twenty-seven-year-old makeup artist from Hollywood, says, "I've tried a lot of kava products and none does a thing for me. What seems to be effective is the liquid extract. A few droppersful under the tongue, and you feel the kava within minutes— calming, euphoric, a marvelous herb. But the taste is horrible. Another option I have found is to mix it in some sort of liquid and then hold my nose and swallow." Ben, from Kansas City, Kansas, agrees, "I didn't have much luck with kava in tea or capsule form, but recently I tried the tincture, and so far it is the most helpful approach to anxiety that I've found—but very costly. I paid ten dollars for a bottle that would last me a week at the recommended dosages."

You can mix the kava tincture in water, milk, soy milk, or juice and ingest it that way. Tinctures work well, but they are very expensive.

TEA

Kava teas are available in health food stores. However, since many of the psychoactive ingredients are fat soluble, most teas are probably not very effective in inducing the type of central nervous system effect that one desires. Although the Pacific natives drink kava tea, most of the time they chew the roots and mix it with saliva, and then coconut milk, which allows the fat-soluble compounds to be more readily available. Then again, everyone has his or her personal preferences, and you may find that you enjoy the tea and it gives you the effect you are looking for.

Because the tea can be bitter, you may want to sweeten it. Stevia is a natural sweetener that takes the bitter edge off kava drinks. See *Stevia: Cooking with Nature's No-Calorie Sweetener* for details.

KAVA PASTE

Some manufactures have kava available as a dark-colored paste. This can be rubbed on sensitive teeth or gums for a numbing effect.

KAVA SPRAY

There's even a spray you can squirt in your mouth. One cinnamon-flavored product claims to have 75 milligrams in the recommended dose.

You may not know exactly how much kavalactones you are getting in the tincture, liquid, or tea. But, as with kava capsules, more important than knowing the exact amount of the active ingredients is how you feel on the product. In addition to experimenting with different brands of products, you may want to try the different forms. I compare this to melatonin. In my experience, I have found that some patients prefer melatonin in the sublingual form, others like the timed-release capsule, and still others like the regular pills. Melatonin tea is another popular option.

HOW LONG CAN I TAKE KAVA?

Kava can be taken occasionally as long as you want. I know individuals who have been using kava off and on all their lives. However, as with many medicines, regular, daily use for more than a few months is discouraged unless it is absolutely necessary. Those who have chronic anxiety can take kava for a few months and then temporarily switch to another medicine. After a break from kava for a few weeks, the herb can be restarted. This way, the potential for any possible long-term side effects is minimized. South Pacific islanders have consumed extracts of the kava root regularly for hundreds of years. Side effects have developed in only regular high-dose users.

WHAT ABOUT TOLERANCE?

As with the use of many medicines that induce relaxation, a concern has been raised that daily high-dose use could lead to kava being ineffective. The brain may adapt to kava exposure and build a resistance to it. In one mouse study, high doses of the liquid extract were able to induce tolerance within a short period of time; however, kava resin was not able to induce tolerance (Duffield 1991). Lower dosages of kava were also not able to induce tolerance. Dr. P. H. Duffield, of the School of Physiology and Pharmacology at the University of New South Wales in Australia, says, "It appears difficult to induce the development of physiological or learned tolerance to kava resin in mice." Practically speaking, this means that reasonable doses of kava used regularly by humans, with occasional breaks, will have little chance of inducing tolerance.

The longest kava has been given daily to humans in a well-controlled study is twenty-four weeks (Volz 1997). No significant side effects were reported. However, at this point, it is still best to limit your regular intake to no longer than six months, unless, of course, a health care practitioner is supervising you and believes other options are not available.

13

INTERVIEWS WITH KAVA EXPERTS

Lise Alschuler, N.D., is Chair of the Botanical Medicine Department at Bastyr University in Seattle, Washington. She regularly uses botanical medicines in her clinical practice.

Kava is a good option for the therapy of anxiety. I prescribe a capsule three times a day to patients who have anxiety, but I prefer the tincture. The tincture is a 1:5 concentration, and I prescribe 2.5 milliliters three times a day.

In my experience, more than half of my patients have some relief with kava. There have been no side effects, because I use low dosages. The longest I have had a patient on kava is six months. This patient has not had side effects. However, I normally prefer to use kava for shorter periods of time.

As to insomnia, kava can be combined with valerian and other herbs. In some cases, I add kava to a headache formula, especially if the headache is of muscle tension origin.

I would like to caution people that kava can be misused. There is a potential for toxicity on high doses if used regularly.

As to valerian root, it has more of a sedative action and is more appropriate for sleep. If a high dose is taken during the day, a person can be lethargic. Kava, in contrast, can reduce anxiety without the lethargy.

Logan Chamberlain, Ph.D., is publisher of *Herbs for Health* magazine.

I use kava at the office sometimes if I'm expecting some kind of stress. It allows me to function without anger or pressure. A calm feeling comes on, but mental alertness stays sharp. If a large dose is ingested, I find myself withdrawing from stimulation and becoming introspective. I have taken ten times the recommended dose without problems. I don't think kava, though, provides any psychological insights.

Gary Friedman is an experienced kava user for more than three decades. He uses kava at least once a week in various forms and understands many of the subtle nuances of this psychoactive Pacific herb. Mr. Friedman is the co-owner of Cosmopolitan Trading/Kava Kompani located in both Seattle, Washington, and in the Republic of Vanuatu. The company supplies premium raw kava to the herbal supplement industry.

Essentially, kava relaxes the body while leaving the mind alert. The effects of fresh kava are very different from dried kava and kava extracts. Fresh kava—particularly the more potent varieties from Vanuatu—prepared in the traditional water-infused manner has psychoactive effects and is more intoxicating. Although I enjoy fresh kava mostly to enhance social settings, I prefer kava extracts for relieving stress or anxiety and helping me to sleep.

The traditional time to consume kava in the Pacific islands is at sunset. Likewise, I generally take larger doses of kava extracts at the end of the day or small amounts about one-half hour before going to sleep. Although some people claim to have dreamless sleep on kava, I find that it produces a deep sleep with highly vivid dreams and that I'm totally refreshed upon awakening. However, if you take too much kava, your mind may become overactive and you may have difficulty sleeping.

What really matters in choosing a kava product is knowing which brands use the right source materials (i.e., quality root) and properly extract the entire spectrum of the kavalactones. As a practical matter, I don't find much difference between various delivery methods of extracts, whether they be liquid, capsule, tablet or spray forms. In liquid form, however, one must be careful to choose a true extract over a tincture. Anybody can make a tincture by simply soaking ground dried herb or mascerated fresh herb in consumable alcohol, whereas it takes much more sophisticated equipment and methods to make a proper extract. Although there is no standard extraction method in the supplement industry, must processes require the use of toxic solvents under heat and their subsequent removal with extreme vacuum. Powders (for tablets and capsules) are then created by laying the extract onto the spent botanical material or an inert carrier. Because of the cost and expertise involved, only a couple of dozen companies actually manufacture extracts for the entire industry.

All kava is cultivated, as the plant is not capable of sexually reproducing on its own. There are about 120 species, each with a different kavalactone profile. Traditionally, and even now, these different species are mostly identified through their physical characteristics—such as shape and color of the plant, its taste and odor, etc.—by experienced cultivators. If the cultivators like a particular plant, they harvest the root and take cuttings from plant stems to start new plants. There have recently been attempts to harvest the leaves of the plants only, but this has so far proven unsuccessful, as the leaves contain a much lower amount and lesser profile of kavalactones and the plants die after two or three harvesting cycles. In the islands of Vanuatu, which is generally considered the original source of kava, various parts of the plant are used in traditional medicine as external poultices for topical anesthetic and anti-fungal effects and ingested to combat pain, urinary tract infections and certain venereal diseases. However, kava is most widely used in ceremonial or social contexts and to facilitate conflict resolution. In the South Pacific, kava is offered as a greeting to honored guests. Kava bars abound—dimly lit places where drinkers gather nightly to consume the beverage of choice and spend hour after hour of animated yet hushed-toned discussion without altercations ever occurring. Islanders have recognized that when kava is consumed, the first thing that goes is aggression—even to the extent that certain highly potent cultivars (know as 'War Kava') are reserved for when tribes or villages are about to go to battle. The would-be combatants consume the kava together and find themselves wondering what's to fight about. Chiefs—the island equivalent of congressmen and senators—quaff mild varieties of kava while considering a plethora of issues for endless hours and find themselves agreeing on just about everything. Extracts of kava are a Western innovation. The dry skin lesion, known as kava dermopathy, and skin discoloration, which have been known to result from consumption of fresh kava, do not appear to occur with the extract. Perhaps the dermothapy is due to the tannins contained in fresh kava; it's also possible that flavokavains produce the discoloration. In any case, one has to ingest copious quantities of kava to produce either or both of these conditions, which requires drinking bowls of fresh kava all day long. There are people on the islands—usually termed 'kava heads'—who do just that. The effect of kava that a person experiences depends on multiple factors, including the particular species and parts of the plant used, the age of the plant (kavalactone potency increases as the plant ages), the extraction process used, the delivery system (such as tincture or other liquid extract, paste extract as contained in soft gels, capsules from powder extract, the new lyposprays, etc.), formulations with other herbals, the metabolic rate of different carriers, the setting of the experience, combined with the very significant factors of dosage and each individual's unique metabolism and . . . well, you can begin to see the endless permutations and possibilities that will influence a person's kava experience. While the U. S. herbal supplement industry and European over-the-counter pharmaceutical trade are primarily marketing kava as a medication for stress, anxiety and mild depression, some other interesting new kava products are currently being developed, such as kava ointments for insect bites, kava chewing gum for minor toothache, kava toothpaste for people with sensitive gums, kava lozenges for sore throat, etc. Kava is even being experimented with as a possible calmative for violent prison inmates and children with attention deficit disorders.

Ironically, this herb that has been used for more than three millennia by islanders who are considered primitive by western standards, may turn out to be the ultimate antidote to the increasingly troubled western world of the 90's. Although a relative novice [compared to those islanders] in travelling kava's psychoactive complexities, my personal conclusion is that kava used in proper moderation is a safe, non-addictive substance of possibly unlimited physical and psychic benefits.

Bob Martin D.C., is a chiropractic doctor and host on KFYI-AM 910, a radio station in Phoenix, Arizona.

Kava works well for anxiety, I recommend it to be used usually toward mid to late afternoon. Patients tell me that kava makes them feel like they are on a small dose of a tranquilizer but without the fuzziness. The thinking process is still clear.

Jan McBarron, M.D., is board certified in preventive medicine and practices in Columbus, Georgia.

I take two kava pills half an hour before going to the dentist. It helps me relax. This herb works great for anxiety. The majority of users respond to it. I believe it is a great alternative to Xanax. At least half of my patients are able to give up Xanax.

Rob McCaleb is president and founder of Herb Research Foundation in Boulder, Colorado.

Q: There have been cases of kava dermopathy in the Polynesian Islands from heavy drinkers of this root. Have you heard of any skin problems associated with kava in the U.S.?

A: I attended a symposium on kava recently. None of the researchers presented any evidence that users in the U.S. or Europe have had this problem. Perhaps it's associated with a compound in the fresh root? We're not sure.

Q: The kava drunk by Polynesians is the water extract of the root. What about the capsules sold in the U.S. Would they have a different content of active ingredients?

A: Probably. But let's keep in mind that many fat-soluble compounds do make it in liquids. For instance, many aromatic oils in teas find themselves in the liquid. I would suspect, with our current extraction techniques, that the capsules sold in vitamin stores would have more active ingredients than just drinking the liquid.

Yadhu N. Singh, Ph.D., is Professor of Pharmacology, College of Pharmacy, South Dakota State University, in Brookings.

Q: Does kava cause alertness or sedation? My experience with the capsules is that they make me feel more alert.

A: Most of the past literature on kava was based on the beverage. I was born and raised in Fiji, and I am personally very familiar with kava drinking. Most novice drinkers notice the sedation from kava after the second or third bowl. And hours later they eventually fall into a deep sleep. Experienced users of kava don't notice the sedation as much. The taste of kava is not that pleasing. Drinking this herb, just like drinking certain types of alcohol, is an acquired taste. Initially people may not like the feeling of numbness that comes on the tongue.

Q: I read in a health magazine that leaves and stems of the kava plant are also used. Is this true?

A: Traditionally only the roots and stems of the plant are generally used.

Q: Do you see any cause for concern with kava becoming more popular. Could it be abused?

A: Abuse of any supplement or herb is possible. Whenever a particular psychoactive compound is transported from one culture to another culture, certain people may not know how to handle it. This occurred with the Australian Aborigines who did not have the ceremonial restraints of kava use.

Terry Willard, Ph.D., an experienced herbalist, is president of Wild Rose College of Natural Healing in Calgary, Canada. He started using kava in 1978. He occasionally uses kava to induce calmness and relaxation.

The effects most people notice include a reduction of anxiety without interference in thinking. People are able to drive without problems, unless an extremely high dose is ingested. Some people find that it helps with fibromyalgia. Cystitis (inflammation of the bladder) is another medical condition where it could be helpful, since kava has some analgesic properties.

The effects normally last four to six hours. When I take it, I notice it within a few minutes. I've been to kava parties where the discussion became deep as a consequence of people using it.

One day I took 4,000 milligrams of the extract, containing 1,200 milligrams of kavalactones. I didn't feel any toxicity or symptoms of overdose.

14

CAUTIONS AND SIDE EFFECTS

As a rule, side effects from the use of kava are significantly less frequent than those from many psychoactive pharmaceutical medicines. However, no herb that has psychoactive and physiological properties can be completely benign.

Symptoms occasionally mentioned by kava users include mild dizziness, insomnia, nausea, and gastrointestinal disturbances. Headaches are infrequent. These symptoms generally occur on high dosages taken at one time. Sandy, a fifty-year-old secretary from Los Angeles, says, "I took five kava pills each containing 70 milligrams of kavalactones on an empty stomach in the morning. Within a half hour I felt nauseated and slightly dazed. The day before, I had taken three pills. On this lower dosage I experienced a relaxed, mellow feeling that lasted about four hours." Denise, who's thirty-four years old, had a similar reaction. "I took three kava pills each containing 99 milligrams of kavalactones, and within an hour I felt nauseated and weak. This feeling lasted about an hour, and then I felt fine again." If you require a high dose of kava to feel an effect, your best option is to take a pill several times a day instead of taking multiple pills at one time.

Heavy consumption of kava is associated with a skin disorder consisting of a scaly rash and eye irritation. Members of Captain Cook's South Pacific expeditions observed these skin signs more than two centuries ago.

In 1990, Dr. P. Ruze of Dartmouth Medical School in Hanover, New Hampshire, interviewed and examined two hundred male kava drinkers with skin changes living in the island of Tonga (Ruze 1990). All of these individuals were heavy drinkers and consumed kava daily. Out of the two hundred drinkers, twenty-nine had significant skin changes. In addition to itchy, dry skin, some had eye irritation. These twenty-nine were randomized to receive either 100 milligrams of nicotinamide (a form of niacin, a B vitamin) or placebo daily for three weeks. The reason this B vitamin was chosen was that the skin lesions looked similar to a pellagra, a severe form of niacin deficiency. After three weeks, there was no major change in the skin condition. Apparently, heavy daily kava consumption causes a scaly rash that is not due to niacin deficiency. The reason for this skin condition still eludes scientists, but some researchers think that kava extracts may possibly interfere with cholesterol metabolism (Norton 1994).

Very heavy consumption of kava also harms the liver, heart, and lungs. The health status of thirty-nine kava users and thirty-four nonusers in a coastal Aboriginal community in Arnhem Land, Australia, was evaluated by researchers from Menzies School of Health Research (Mathews 1988). Twenty respondents were very heavy users (about 60 grams a day of the crude root powder), fifteen respondents were heavy users (about 40 grams a day), and four were occasional users (15 grams a day). These kava users were more likely to complain of poor health and a "puffy" face, and they were more likely to have a typical scaly rash. Their knee reflexes were slightly slower. In addition, very heavy users weighed 20 percent less than the nonusers and had elevated liver enzymes. This indicates that excessive kava consumption on a daily basis for prolonged periods can cause harm to the liver. These types of side effects have not yet been reported in Western countries.

There have been rare reports in the medical literature of an allergic reaction to kava extract (Suss 1996). A high dose of kava in certain individuals can lead to skin reactions and disturbances in coordination. Vision can sometimes be temporarily affected (Garner 1985). In one patient, the ingestion of a kava drink led to a reduced near-point accommodation, making it slightly more difficult to focus on near objects, such as reading a book. This subject also had dilated pupils. My own experience with kava has been slightly different. I notice a very mild clarity of vision an hour or two after ingesting a capsule. The effect is subtle. Patients I have prescribed kava to have also reported this visual enhancement. Even auditory enhancement has been reported by a few users.

One of the positive effects of kava ingestion is muscle relaxation. However, when excessive dosages are used, this can lead to temporary muscle incoordination.

As the popularity of kava grows, and more and more people use this herb, we may discover side effects not previously reported in the medical literature. If other side effects are found, I plan to post them on my Internet site (http://www.raysahelian.com).

Also keep in mind that medicines to treat anxiety can have very unpleasant side effects. For instance, a certain category of medicines called tricyclics, used to treat depression and anxiety, can have anticholinergic effects of dry mouth and dilated pupils, along with inducing cardiac rhythm disturbances. Thus far studies have not shown kava to have any significant effect on the heart when used in the proper dosages.

THE INTOXICATED AUSTRALIAN ABORIGINE

A report in the *Medical Journal of Australia* in August of 1997 begins, "Over the past 15 years, kava has been consumed (often in quantities far exceeding those in ceremonial use) in some Aboriginal communities in Arnhem Land in Northern Territory. We report a case of an acute neurological syndrome associated with heavy kava consumption.

"A 27-year-old Aboriginal Australian man from Arnhem Land presented to our hospital three times with generalized choreoathetosis [sudden, irregular jerking movements of muscles] due to kava ingestion. During the episodes, he has severe choreoathetosis involving his limbs, trunk, neck, facial musculature and even tongue. His level of consciousness is unimpaired and the remainder of the examination is normal. On each occasion, his symptoms largely settled following the administration of intravenous diazepam [Valium], and within 12 hours he was asymptomatic [without symptoms] on examination, indicating an acute intoxication syndrome."

During these emergency evaluations, the examining doctors did not find any major abnormalities in blood tests except for some liver enzyme elevations (indicative of liver irritation by the excessive kava drinking). Temporary liver enzyme elevations can also occur when people drink a large amount of alcohol.

Overconsumption of any supplement, herb, nutrient, food, or hormone is not advised. This is also true of kava. It is an herb that has medical benefits if used appropriately, but it should not be used excessively.

KAVA AND ALCOHOL

As we all know, alcohol doesn't mix too well with many sedatives and sleep medicines. In mouse studies, the combination of kava and alcohol has shown to be additive (Jamieson

1990). Alcohol increased the effect of kava. The researchers state, "This interaction of kava and alcohol has important clinical and social consequences since, in contrast to traditional usage, kava is now often taken in conjunction with alcoholic drinks." However, another study did not find any untoward reactions when kava and alcohol were combined (Herberg 1993).

A dose of kavalactones less than 100 milligrams combined with a small glass of wine or less than six ounces of beer should not present any significant interaction. But everyone is different, and if you are sensitive to alcohol, I urge caution. I have taken a kava capsule in the evening and then had a glass of wine with dinner with no untoward consequences. In fact, my mind stayed sharp. However, alcohol is deceptive. One or two drinks may be just fine, but problems could arise after the third or fourth glass.

It is also possible that kava, since it causes initial alertness, can partially counteract the sedating effects of alcohol. When it comes to the combination of kava and alcohol, it is very difficult to predict what will happen since each of us reacts differently not only to kava but also to alcohol. Therefore, if you plan to use both concurrently, take very low dosages initially to see how this combination influences you.

KAVA AND LIBIDO

I am frequently asked whether kava has any effect on sex drive or sexual enjoyment. The influence of kava on libido has not been reported in the medical literature. From my personal observations and discussions with users, kava does not seem to have a strong influence on the sexual response one way or the other. It is possible that the sedating properties of kava subsequent to the initial alertness can make one less energetic or interested in the pursuit of sex. Another point to consider is that kava has some anesthetic, or painkilling, properties and could theoretically decrease the sensitivity of the sexual organs.

On the other hand, if anxiety is distracting or inhibiting a person from feeling intimate, it is possible that the relaxation induced by kava could help him or her become more in the mood for lovemaking.

IS KAVA ADDICTIVE?

Until the 1980s, the Australian Aborigines had no contact with kava. Missionaries from the

Polynesian islands who came to their communities introduced the plant to them (Cawte 1985). Some Aboriginal leaders, having visited the Polynesian islands, were impressed by the kava ceremony and recommended this plant as a substitute for alcohol. Unfortunately, certain Aborigines, unfamiliar with the traditional ceremonial use of kava for special circumstances, started drinking it regularly. Thus, kava partially replaced alcohol, and an epidemic of kava abuse became prevalent among the Aborigines in Northern Australia. Although kava abuse does not lead to aggressiveness and violence, it can lead to apathy and domestic neglect.

My clinical experience with kava does not indicate that it is physically addictive. However, it does have the potential to be habit-forming in a minority of individuals who are prone to substance misuse. If kava were not available, these individuals would most likely overuse alcohol or other mood-altering substances.

When kava is prescribed for daily use for therapeutic purposes, it should be limited to no more than six months.

WHAT ABOUT WITHDRAWAL SYMPTOMS?

One of the serious shortcomings of benzodiazepine antianxiety agents such as Valium and Xanax is the potential for withdrawal symptoms on abrupt discontinuation after regular use. The symptoms of withdrawal include agitation, restlessness, insomnia, excessive anxiety, and even seizures. There are no reports in the medical literature of any serious withdrawal reactions when kava usage is stopped. In the twenty-five-week study of kava administration by Dr. Volz discussed in Chapter 4, no withdrawal symptoms were observed when the volunteers stopped their kava medication.

CAN I DRIVE A CAR WHILE TAKING KAVA?

Although kava does not, in the prescribed dosages, produce the mental disorientation and slowing that benzodiazepines (Valium) and other tranquilizers do, caution is still advised. I recommend that the first few times you try kava you do so when you're not expected to drive a car or operate heavy machinery. If you discover that kava does not interfere with your mental clarity, then it is reasonable to drive a car while taking kava. Most users find that kava actually makes them more alert and aware. Furthermore, the mild relaxation that comes from kava could potentially make a person less aggressive on the highway and even more tolerant when encountering traffic congestion.

Keep in mind, though, that excessive consumption or an overdose of kava can perhaps lead to muscle uncoordination, and thus, as common sense would advise, it is not safe to be behind a wheel of a car when intoxicated. Furthermore, although kava can initially lead to alertness and stimulation, it could potentially, many hours later, lead to relaxation and drowsiness. Therefore, if you have a long car drive ahead of you, kava may not be the best medicine to take. Caffeine is an option, and so are the amino acids tyrosine and phenylalanine, which are known to enhance alertness. Pregnenolone also enhances alertness and awareness and can be taken at a dose of 10 milligrams when expecting to drive for prolonged periods.

CAUTION

There are certain individuals who probably should not use kava unless it's specifically recommended by a medical professional. Be very cautious in using kava if:

- You have Parkinson's disease. Kava could possibly block dopamine receptors in the brain, and Parkinson's disease needs dopamine. In fact, L-dopa is a medicine prescribed to those who have Parkinson's disease. Another medicine given to these patients is selegiline (Eldepryl, deprenyl), which elevates dopamine levels in the brain.
- You are severely depressed and you are trying to self-medicate. It is best to have a medical professional help you with your therapy.
- You are pregnant or nursing. You should avoid kava unless recommended by a physician when other ways to reduce anxiety are not available or are not appropriate.

If you are elderly, or medically very frail, you should be very careful anytime you take supplements. Always take the lowest amount. This could even mean opening a capsule and taking a third of a dose initially. If you tolerate this low dose, then the next day you can take half a dose, and continue increasing it daily.

Of course, anytime you have a coexisting medical condition, or are on other medicines, a health care practitioner should supervise you when adding supplements.

There have been rare cases of acute dystonic reactions on kava (Schelosky 1995). A dystonic reaction is a sudden spasm of a part of the body, including the neck, trunk, or tongue. The doses reported were generally more than 100 milligrams of kavalactones, and all of these rare cases were reported in Europe.

Of course, as mentioned previously, kava is not intended to be used on a regular basis and in a high dose for long periods since it can potentially lead to the side effects discussed on previous pages.

CAN A URINE DRUG TEST TELL IF I'VE TAKEN KAVA?

A routine urine drug test usually checks for alcohol, cocaine, marijuana, narcotics, steroids, and certain prescription sedatives and painkillers. To test for kava, a special request must be submitted to the testing laboratory, since evaluating for kava metabolites in blood or urine is not a routine procedure. A specific laboratory test, known as gas chromatography–

mass spectrometry, can determine levels of metabolites of kavalactones and yangonin (Duffield 1989).

Kava ingestion is perfectly legal. There would be a concern, though, if excessive amounts were consumed that would interfere with your ability to operate machinery or drive a vehicle.

15
VALERIAN

Valerian is a plant widely distributed in North America, Europe, and Asia, growing wild in woods and along riverbanks. At least a couple of hundred species of this plant have been categorized, and the most commonly recognized species is called *Valeriana officinalis*. Known to the Greeks from the time of Hippocrates, this herb has been used since the Middle Ages for nervous disturbances affecting the gastrointestinal system and for sleep (Holzl 1989). Its popularity grew in the nineteenth century when it became used more frequently for its relaxing effects. It was even used during World War I to combat shell shock (Wolman 1972). Valerian remained in the American and English pharmacopoeias until the middle of the twentieth century, when it gradually lost popularity as the barbiturates and benzodiazepines were discovered. It was dropped from *The National Formulary* in 1950. The root, where the active ingredients are found, has an unpleasant aroma, which has slightly interfered with its popularity. The fresh herb does not have much of a smell. This smell develops with time due to the enzymatic breakdown of the compounds in the herb (Houghton 1988).

Valerian has been available in Europe under several trade names, including Euvegal, Valmane, Valdispert forte, Nutrasleep, and Biral.

WHAT'S IN VALERIAN?

The root of the plant contains three distinctive types of compounds: volatile oils (sequiterpenes such as valerenic acid, valernal, and valenol), valepotriates, and a small number of alkaloids. The valepotriates appear to be the most active of these chemicals (Houghton 1988), although water extracts, which do not contain valepotriates, have also been shown to have sleep-inducing effects (Leathwood 1982, 1985). There are dozens of chemicals in valerian, and many have not yet been fully identified. A standardized extract containing three valepotriates is marketed in Germany under the trade name Valmane. It consists of 80 percent didrovaltrate, 15 percent valtrate, and 5 percent acevaltrate (Houghton 1988).

The composition and proportion of chemicals in valerian, as with other herbs, depends on a number of factors including the geographical location it is grown, type of soil, age of harvesting, and the season of harvesting.

HOW DOES VALERIAN WORK?

The exact mechanism of action of the different compounds in valerian root has not been fully elicited. Preliminary research indicates that certain compounds in valerian influence some of the same brain receptors as do the benzodiazepine medicines such as Valium and Xanax (Holzl 1989). These receptors are called GABA, which stands for gamma-aminobutyric acid. Activation of GABA receptors leads to relaxation and sleep. In one study, water extracts of valerian stimulated the release of GABA in brain cell synapses, in addition to preventing the reuptake of this inhibitory neurotransmitter (Santos 1994). This simply means that more GABA was present in the brain, leading to sedation. There are probably many other ways that valerian influences brain chemistry. Another study found that valerian actually contains a high amount of the neurotransmitter GABA, which would directly induce sedation (Cavadas 1995). However, GABA can cross the blood-brain barrier only in very high dosages, and it alone cannot account for valerian's sedative effects. Scientists are still in the early learning stages when it comes to uncovering the actions of compounds in the valerian root.

Valerian is not nearly as powerful as many pharmaceutical sedatives or sleep medicines. A study in mice comparing the sedative effects of valerian to diazepam and chlorpromazine showed the herb to have less pronounced effects (Leuschner 1993). The advantage of valerian is that there is less of a concern that overdose would cause serious respiratory depression or even death as would be likely with the benzodiazepines.

Compounds in this herb are also thought to have smooth-muscle-relaxing properties.

VALERIAN FOR INSOMNIA

Several studies over the past two decades have indicated that valerian is useful in both inducing the onset of sleep and in providing a deeper sleep (Leathwood 1982, 1983, 1985). A double-blind, placebo-controlled study done using an aqueous extract of 400 milligrams of valerian done with 128 subjects showed improvements in sleep onset and in sleep quality (Leathwood 1982).

In a more recent study, fourteen elderly poor sleepers received 405 milligrams of a valerian preparation (product name Valdispert) three times a day for a week. The amount of time it took them to fall asleep decreased, and their deep, slow-wave sleep was enhanced (Schulz 1994). REM sleep, also known as the stage where dreams occur, was not affected. This study needs to be interpreted cautiously since the number of subjects was small.

Unlike pharmaceutical sleeping pills that induce grogginess and hangover, valerian does not impair vigilance in the morning to any significant extent (Gerhard 1996). In a study conducted in Basel, Switzerland, valerian and hops were compared to flunitrazepam, a benzodiazepine hypnotic prescribed in Europe. Impairment of performance in the morning was found only on flunitrazepam, not the herbs. The researchers say, "Impairment of vigilance on the morning after ingestion of benzodiazepines, frequently reported and confirmed by our results, constitutes a potential hazard. In this situation, plant remedies such as those examined in this study should be considered as viable alternatives."

I have taken valerian and have noticed that it aids in improving sleep quality. Its effects are not as powerful, and not as consistent, as those of the pharmaceutical sleep medicines. However, I have also noticed that the use of this herb generally does not lead to a feeling of hangover that is associated with the use of pharmaceutical drugs. The highest dose I have tried is eight pills each containing 100 milligrams of the extract (for a total of 800 milligrams). This product was standardized to contain 0.8 percent of valerenic acid. I would say valerian works for me four out of five times. I am currently taking valerian about once a week.

A. E. Smith, age seventy-one, from Bellevue, Washington, says, "Valerian is priceless. I was on the prescription sleeping pill Prosom (estazolam) for three years. I got off Prosom in May of 1997 but found it impossible to sleep without it. Melatonin worked for a while too, but then I discovered I needed to take higher and higher dosages. I've been on valerian for two months now and it works like a charm. I take two 160-milligram capsules, standardized to contain 0.2 percent valerenic acid, about half an hour before bed. There's no grogginess in the morning. If I find the valerian is not enough, and I still have an active mind, then I add about 1 milligram of melatonin. There's been no problem with the combination." Debbie, thirty-eight, from Washington, D.C., agrees. "Valerian is great. One 430 milligram capsule brings on a nice 'calm' within forty-five minutes and I am able to fall asleep easily."

Valerian does not work as consistently for everyone. Denise, a thirty-two-year-old entertainment lawyer, says, "I tried valerian when a girlfriend told me how well it worked for her. Having had a few occasions to use it, I can't say it works all the time. In fact, at times it has made me very wired, and very odd thoughts race through my head. This is the very opposite of the desired effect. But, when I take valerian with melatonin, it works very well. As a side note, I should mention that my cat loves the smell of valerian, She goes nuts when I open the bottle and let her have a whiff, or even when I've just had the capsules in my hand momentarily."

Scott, a thirty-four-year-old actor from Malibu, California, has had a similar experience: "Valerian has a paradoxical effect on me. It causes me to be slightly agitated rather than relaxed."

In addition to a few patients who have reported having worse sleep than normal on valerian, one has noted experiencing restless legs. The reason that some people do not react to valerian, or even feel slightly stimulated, is not known. Perhaps it may be due to different valerian species, or products, having a different set or proportion of chemical constituents. Or perhaps some individuals have a brain chemistry that responds differently to the chemicals in valerian. Another possibility is the timing of the dosage. Perhaps some individuals would respond better taking the valerian capsules, or drinking the tea, several hours before bed as opposed to near bedtime.

VALERIAN FOR ANXIETY

Even though the primary use of valerian is for insomnia, many physicians sometimes recommend it for anxiety. However, the amount of valerian used during the day should be less than the nightly dose since a large dose could potentially make one sleepy during the day, interfering with work performance or driving skills.

Having said this, we should keep in mind that there is a wide range of reactions to valerian. Nancy, a fifty-four-year-old rental leasing agent from Anaheim, California, took a

50-milligram valerian capsule standardized to contain 0.8 percent valeric acid at 10 A.M. in the morning. An hour later, she took a second pill. Instead of being sedated, she actually felt more energized and couldn't stop doing chores around the house. She described the feeling as being restless. However, she started feeling sleepy about 1 P.M. and took a brief nap. Another patient, a thirty-year-old flight attendant, finds that valerian at 50 milligrams induces relaxation without sleepiness. She says, "Valerian works quite well for me in relieving anxiety and nervous tension. I've been taking the alcohol extract on and off for ten years without side effects. I consider this herb a long-term friend."

Kava has been studied much more extensively for the therapy of anxiety than has valerian. You may also want to experiment using small dosages of both herbs as a combination therapy for anxiety. Of course, be sure to seek the help of an experienced health care practitioner whenever you experiment with supplements or the combination of herbs.

VALERIAN MAY HELP YOU WITHDRAW FROM SLEEP DRUGS

A potential area that deserves to be explored is the substitution of valerian for pharmaceutical sleep drugs. One study done on rats showed that valerian therapy eased symptoms of benzodiazepine withdrawal (Andreatini 1994). There is a good possibility that this could also be accomplished in humans if done gradually. For instance, if a person has been taking a particular sleep medicine every night for a few weeks, he or she can substitute valerian one night and monitor the effectiveness of the herb. This would, of course, be done under the guidance of a health care practitioner. If the valerian is helpful, it can be substituted for the drug perhaps twice a week, and then three times a week, and eventually nightly. Another option is also to introduce melatonin for one or two nights a week in place of the valerian, or in place of the sleep drug. My clinical experience and a published medical report indicate the melatonin can be substituted for sleep drugs in certain individuals (Dagan 1997). You have to be cautious, though, whenever you have been on a benzodiazepine sleep drug for prolonged periods. Abrupt cessation of these drugs can potentially lead to serious withdrawal symptoms, including seizures.

ANTISEIZURE PROPERTIES

Two studies conducted on mice have shown that valerian extracts have mild anticonvulsant activity (Dunaev 1987, Leuschner 1993). The clinical significance of these findings in humans is not clear at this time.

MISCELLANEOUS USES

Over the years, valerian root tea and extracts have been recommended for a number of conditions including stomach cramps, irritable bowel, and menstrual cramps. Valerian may have some muscle-relaxing properties in animal tissues (Hazelhoff 1982), but we need actual human trials to determine the effectiveness of valerian in the above disorders.

WHAT'S THE RIGHT DOSAGE?

Generally a dose of 300 to 500 milligrams of the concentrated root extract providing 0.5 to 1 percent of the essential oils (such as valerinic acid) is effective in inducing and maintaining sleep. Some people with stubborn insomnia may require more. Take the valerian one half to two hours before retiring.

Teas are also effective and many companies sell prepackaged tea bags. You can also steep about a teaspoon of the dried roots per cup. Tinctures or liquid extracts are another option. Generally anywhere between 2 to 5 milliliters can help induce sleep. This depends, of course, on the concentration of the tincture and liquid.

It's difficult to give exact dosages since there are hundreds of different compounds on the market. Many of these have been extracted using different methods, and they therefore may contain different amounts and concentrations of the essential oils, valepotriates, and other sedative chemicals.

As for its daytime use in the therapy of anxiety, start with a smaller dose, such as 100 milligrams. The first time you take valerian during the day should preferably be on a weekend when you are not at work or you don't have to drive. This is just in case you happen to be very sensitive to valerian's sedative properties.

HOW SOON DOES IT WORK?

Most users will notice the effects of valerian within an hour, although some obtain the best benefits taking the valerian two to three hours before bed.

Hundreds of valerian products are sold by mail order and in vitamin stores, herb shops, pharmacies, and retail outlets. Some are standardized to contain a particular flavonoid in the herb. There are, though, no universally accepted standardized preparations. Here's a sampling of a few products.

Capsules and Pills

Valerian root capsule 50 milligrams standardized to contain 0.8 percent of valeric acid

Valerian root capsule 160 milligrams standardized to contain 0.2 percent valerenic acid, combined with 80 milligrams of lemon balm

Valerian root capsule 300 milligrams standardized to contain 1 percent valerenic acid

Valerian root capsule, 425 milligrams, nonstandardized

Valerian root capsule, 475 milligrams, nonstandardized

Valerian root capsule, 500 milligrams, nonstandardized

Valerian root capsule, 530 milligrams, non-standardized

Combinations

You can find valerian combined with single herbs, or a combination of several sedating herbs. Often it is combined with passionflower, kava, hops, skullcap, or chamomile. One company has combined 70 milligrams of valerian with 60 milligrams of skullcap, 40 milligrams of passionflower, 40 milligrams of hops, and 40 milligrams of chamomile.

Liquid

Valerian root liquid: Each dropper (1 milliliter) contains 300 milligrams of 1 percent valerenic acid. The liquids are often alcoholic extracts of the valerian root.

Tea

Several brands are available, and these are not standardized. Many of the sedative components of valerian are water-soluble, and thus they would be able to induce sleep (Leathwood 1982, 1985).

HOW OFTEN CAN I USE VALERIAN?

Sleeping pills, whether drugs, herbs, or hormones (such as melatonin), should not be used indefinitely. The underlying cause or causes of the insomnia should be searched for and corrected. However, there are times in almost everyone's life where periods of insomnia or shallow sleep develop, and the temporary use of these supplements can be of tremendous benefit.

Valerian appears to be safe for nightly consumption if limited to a few weeks. It is best to avoid using this herb nightly for prolonged periods of time, such as more than six months, since no long-term studies of continuous use have been published. Another reason not to use it continuously is the possibility of tolerance in certain individuals. Martha, a forty-year-old homemaker, says, "For me, valerian seems to create a tolerance almost immediately, in that it doesn't work well two days in a row and is useless on the third. So I save it for times when I really need the extra push into sleepiness." Martha's quick sensitivity to valerian's tolerance is unusual.

Based on my clinical experience over the years, I prefer not to rely exclusively on any particular medicine for prolonged periods. There may be some components in certain herbs that are not agreeable to our body if regularly ingested for a long time. However, even if a particular herb or medicine has some harmful effects on the body, its occasional use would present no problems since the body has a remarkable ability to detoxify unwanted chemicals. For this reason I feel comfortable in recommending the occasional use of certain herbs for particular medicinal purposes, realizing that the potential gains they provide far outweigh their possible harm. In the case of valerian, I feel that the deep sleep it provides when used occasionally is far more beneficial to the body and brain than the tossing and turning that could result on certain nights without its use.

I also feel that melatonin is a safe hormone to use for sleep if taken occasionally, such as once or twice a week. If you have a stubborn case of insomnia, you can use valerian once or twice a week and also use melatonin once or twice a week. This way, your body is not being exposed to the same substance all the time. Furthermore, there is a potential for tolerance to develop to melatonin and perhaps also the potential to develop tolerance to valerian. By using them infrequently, you can get the benefits of each of these sleep inducers while minimizing any potential problems.

Another option that I have recommended to some patients is the combination of melatonin and valerian. For instance, instead of using 1 milligram of melatonin to induce and maintain sleep, one can use 0.2 to 0.5 milligram combined with a small dose of valerian. One of the side effects of high-dose melatonin use is vivid dreaming, which can be enjoyable if pleasant or, if unpleasant, a nightmare. By decreasing the dose of the melatonin, the potential for side effects is reduced, while maintaining good sleep architecture with the valerian combination.

WHAT ABOUT SIDE EFFECTS?

These are uncommon in the dosages normally consumed. One side effect reported is stomach upset. Anecdotally, a small number of people have reported feeling restless legs overnight. Large doses may, in some susceptible individuals, cause restlessness, tiredness the next day, and headaches.

The interaction of valerian with alcohol, barbiturates, benzodiazepines, and other sedatives has not been officially studied. However, it is always best to be extracautious when combining more than one sedative. The effects could very well be additive.

A COLLEGE STUDENT OVERDOSES

Dr. Leanna Willey, of the Department of Pediatrics at the University of Rochester School of Medicine in Rochester, New York, published a report in 1995 describing the case of an eighteen-year-old college student who was brought to the emergency room three hours after ingesting forty to fifty capsules of valerian. Her intent was to commit suicide. Each capsule contained 470 milligrams powdered valerian root, and her total reported dose was therefore about 20 grams.

Thirty minutes after ingesting this massive amount of valerian, the student experienced fatigue, abdominal cramps, chest tightness, tremor of the hands and feet, and lightheadedness. A physical exam in the emergency room found her vital signs, such as blood pressure and heart rate, to be relatively normal. She had mild pupil dilation and slight tremor in the hands. The EKG (electrocardiogram), blood count and chemistry, and liver enzymes were all normal. She was given activated charcoal to absorb the valerian in her stomach and admitted to the hospital where her symptoms resolved within twenty-four hours. Dr. Willey concludes, "A 20 gram valerian overdose in an adult thus appears benign, supporting previous reports that valerian has a low order of toxicity."

USE IN PREGNANCY

No formal human studies are available evaluating valerian in pregnancy or lactation. Back in 1994, a study was conducted in Brazil assessing the effects of valerian on pregnant rats. A thirty-day oral administration of valepotriates did not induce any major changes in the offspring. The researchers conclude, "Orally given doses of valepotriates were innocuous to pregnant rats and their offspring."

In cases of severe insomnia during pregnancy, a physician has to use his or her best judgment to determine whether the occasional use of valerian to induce a deeper sleep is warranted. Perhaps a deep sleep is a better alternative to a fitful, restless night.

In cases of severe insomnia necessitating the use of a sleep-inducing agent, my opinion as a physician is that valerian is a good alternative to benzodiazepine drugs. The use of melatonin during pregnancy has also not been evaluated, but I suspect that a low dose of 0.2

to 0.5 milligram used no more than once a week should be tolerated well.

Evaluating the full safety of valerian or melatonin in the therapy of insomnia during pregnancy will be a difficult challenge due to obvious medicoethical limitations. No one should use valerian or melatonin when pregnant or nursing without first consulting their health care practitioner.

IS VALERIAN ADDICTIVE?

There seems to be no evidence that the use of this herb is physically addictive. However, just as any supplement, hormone, or herb that induces a noticeable effect, valerian can potentially be habit-forming in certain individuals.

PERSONAL STORIES

Valerian is great. I take it about two hours before bed. What's even better is a combination. I take a pill that contains valerian root, passionflower, magnesium and calcium. It's an amazing combination.—MN, thirty-three, Baltimore, Maryland

I've been using valerian root for about six months now and I love it! It doesn't have the side effects that I was getting taking [a tricyclic antidepressant]. Being a heavy person, I take two at supper and another two at bedtime. I'm sleeping much better this way, and it does help get me relief from [severe] aches at night. I get that much-needed rest that helps me to cope with the day-to-day pain I have to deal with.—JE, thirty-six, Memphis, Tennessee

SUMMARY

The occasional use of valerian, whether in capsule, tea, or tincture, is effective as a sleep aid for many individuals, particularly the elderly. However, a few individuals have a paradoxical reaction to this herb and find themselves slightly more alert.

If you suffer from chronic insomnia, have a medical evaluation to rule out any serious cause of this problem. The next step is to find nonmedicinal ways to treat the problem through exercise and proper sleep habits (See Chapter 10 for suggestions). If you still can't sleep, then the temporary use of valerian is justified.

The chronic use of valerian is not recommended at this time since we don't know the effects of regular, nightly use for prolonged periods. However, if you do need to take a sleeping aid on a regular basis, you could alternate taking valerian, melatonin, 5-hydroxytryptophan, hops, passionflower, and some of the other herbs discussed in this book. This way, you won't be exposing your system to the same chemicals all the time, and this would minimize any potential problems, including the possible development of tolerance. I use valerian tea about once a week and melatonin about once a week. If I need help other nights, I use a combination of chamomile, passionflower, and hops. In fact, you may find, through trial and error, a specific combination of herbs that suits you best. Some individuals find the combinations much more effective than the single herbs alone. The occasional use of a pharmaceutical sleeping pill could also be justified.

16
HOPS

The hop plant is known by the scientific name of *Humulus lupulus*. It's a climbing vine of the hemp family with conelike fruits known as hops. It has grown wild since ancient times in Europe, Asia, and America. For the past millennium, hops have been used in the brewing of beer, contributing a desirable bitter flavor. Early on, it was discovered that hop pickers in the field tired easily, apparently from the transfer of some resin to their mouths during the picking.

HISTORICAL USES OF HOPS

Traditionally, hops have been used as sedatives, antibacterials, and aids in digestive disorders. The young shoots of the plant were eaten as a vegetable, and the dried cones were used for their slightly narcotic and sedative effects in the therapy of aches and pains (Haas 1995).

WHAT'S IN HOPS?

In addition to flavonoids, a number of resins, commonly termed weak acids, are found in hops, including humulene, humulone, lupulin, and colupulone (Simpson 1992, Verschuere 1992).

HOPS AND SLEEP

Whenever I write about supplements and herbs, I take them myself and also prescribe them to patients. Additionally, I have a few close friends who enjoy trying the new supplements and herbs I write about and like to give me their feedback. One morning at 10 A.M., I gave Geraldine, a fifty-year-old friend, two capsules of hops. She didn't know what the capsules contained and what their effects would be, if any. An hour later, she said, "You know what, whatever you gave me is making me tranquil and sleepy. I feel like going to bed and lying down. Are these pills supposed to make me feel this way?" An hour later, her sleepiness had partially worn off and she reported being relaxed and calm.

Most patients who take capsules of hops do feel a slight sedation. They have been traditionally used to treat insomnia and to ease tension and anxiety. I have taken capsules of hops in the evening on several occasions and found them consistently to have sedative and hypnotic properties. Hops have not received as much attention as valerian, but I think they will gradually become more popular.

HOW IS IT AVAILABLE?

Capsules containing hops are sold in a variety of dosages. A recent visit to a vitamin store revealed 150 milligrams of hops standardized to contain 5 percent of humulene, and 150 milligrams of hops standardized to contain 5 percent of bitter acids and 4 percent of flavonoids.

You can also use hops in a tea form by adding a teaspoon of the dried hops flowers to boiling water. Tinctures of hops are available; follow the instructions on the label. Generally, one or two capsules of hops, or a dose of 1 to 5 milliliters of the tincture, are taken an hour or two before bed.

You may also take hops during the day as a

sedative if you are very alert or anxious. In this case, half of the hypnotic (sleep-inducing) dose is enough.

Many sedative herbal products include hops along with other herbs such as chamomile, valerian, and passionflower. These are fine to take; however, the dosages rarely are listed on the bottle. Therefore, you will not know the exact amounts you are ingesting. If a particular product is effective, though, the exact dosage content is really not that important to know.

OTHER PROPERTIES OF HOPS

Humulone, one of the bitters in hops, has inhibitory activity against the tumor-promoting effect of a chemical known as 12-O-tetradecanoylphorbol-13-acetate when applied to the skin (Yasukawa 1995). It also inhibited arachidonic acid-induced inflammatory ear edema in mice. A study done at the Showa College of Pharmaceutical Sciences in Tokyo showed humulone to induce cell death in a certain type of leukemia cell line (Tobe 1997).

The essential oils as well as solvent extracts were isolated from the cones of various hop plants (Langezaal 1992). These showed activity against gram-positive bacteria *Bacillus subtilis* and *Staphylococcus aureus* and the fungus *Trichophyton mentagrophytes* but no activity against the gram-negative bacterium *Escherichia coli* and the yeast *Candida albicans*.

"Beer Hops May Help Prevent Cancer," was a newswire report distributed by Associated Press in March of 1998. According to the article, Oregon State University scientists found that some of the flavonoids in hops, particulary xanthohumol, help enhance the effect of a class of enzymes, called quinone reductase, that block cancer-causing substances that already have been activated in cells. Dr. Donald Buhler, the lead scientist, is quoted saying, "We treated human breast, colon and ovarian cells that were cancerous with concentrations (of flavonoids) that were not harmful to normal cells and found that some of the hops flavonoids were toxic to cancer cells." His findings were reported in Seattle at the annual meeting of the international Society of Toxicology.

CAUTION

Excessive dosages are not recommended for those who are depressed. It also is best to avoid high doses during the day, since the sedation could interfere with work performance and driving. Significant side effects with hops have not been reported in the medical literature.

SUMMARY

Hops has sedative qualities that are stronger than chamomile and passionflower and somewhat similar in strength to valerian. Hops can be used alone at night to induce sleep or can be combined with other sedative herbs. As with other herbs discussed in this book, regular, nightly use for prolonged periods is not recommended. The occasional use of hops is certainly justified as an alternative to sleep-inducing medicines. In preliminary laboratory studies, hops have been found to have some antigerm and antitumor abilities, but the clinical significance of these findings is currently not known.

17

PASSIONFLOWER

Passionflower (*Passiflora incarnata*) is a well-known medicinal plant native to America's hot tropical areas. The aerial parts have been traditionally used in America for the treatment of anxiety, nervousness, and neural pain (Brasseur 1984).

WHAT'S IN PASSIONFLOWER?

The main chemical constituents of this plant are flavonoids, such as vitexin, isovitexin, orientin, kampferol, apigenin (chamomile also contains apigenin), vicenin, lucenin, and swertisin (Lutomski 1960, Quercia 1978, Rahman 1997). In addition, there are several indole alkaloids such as harman, harmin, harmalin, and harmol (Lohdelink 1974).

PASSIONFLOWER AND SLEEP

The administration of extract of passionflower to mice decreased anxious behavior, decreased activity, and led to a sleepy state, indicating that this herb does have sedative properties (Soulimani 1997). The water extract was more effective than the alcoholic extract, suggesting that the active sedative chemicals in passionflower are most likely to be present when the herb is drunk as a tea.

You can drink passionflower tea about one or two hours before bed. It can also be combined with some of the other sedative herbs discussed in this book.

HOW IS IT AVAILABLE?

Passionflower is available in capsules, tincture, and tea. One product contains 250 milligrams of the flower standardized to 4 percent flavonoids, particularly isovitexin.

OTHER PROPERTIES OF PASSIONFLOWER

Historically, passionflower has been used to treat neuralgia, convulsions, and anxiety. Human studies evaluating the role of passion-flower in these conditions is very limited.

SIDE EFFECTS

No significant side effects from the ingestion of moderate amounts of passionflower have been reported in the medical literature. Very large amounts, especially when combined with other relaxing herbs or medicines, could potentially induce excessive sedation or altered consciousness (Solbakken 1997).

Taking a high dose of passionflower during the day is not recommended. Brittany, a forty-five-year-old, took eight capsules of passion-flower in the morning. She reports, "I felt a little tired a couple of hours later. The rest of the day, I felt anxious, irritable, impatient, and continued being tired. I usually go to the gym after work. However, I opted to lie in bed and watch TV. Next time, I'm going to take the passionflower at nighttime."

One morning I took eight capsules of pas-sionflower at about 10 A.M. to test for myself if this herb has any sedative properties. I did notice feeling sleepy at about 1 P.M. An hour later I took a half-hour nap. Thereafter, I was refreshed and alert.

SUMMARY

Passionflower has mild sedative properties and can be used occasionally to induce sleep. The various flavonoids present in the herb could also have beneficial health properties. You most often find passionflower combined with other sedative herbs either in teas or capsules.

As a rule, it may be a good idea to take more than one sedative herb in combination with others, since each one may be too weak to work well on its own. You can take passionflower combined with chamomile, hops, or valerian.

18
CHAMOMILE

Chamomile, a plant of the daisy family, has long been used in folk medicine to treat a variety of disorders. The dried flower heads were brewed to make a tea and used for gastrointestinal symptoms, minor infections, certain skin disorders, and insomnia, especially in children.

There are two main species of chamomile, German (*Matricaria recutita* or *Matricaria chamomilla*) and Roman (*Anthemis nobilis* or *Chamaemelum nobile*). The majority of the studies published with chamomile used the German type, which currently comprises most of the chamomile products available in the U.S. However, you occasionally find the Roman type sold in vitamin stores.

Europeans have used chamomile for centuries. German physicians often recommend pharmaceutical brands called Kamillosan or Perkamillon, mostly for indigestion and ulcers.

WHAT'S IN CHAMOMILE?

All the herbs discussed in this book contain several compounds that have therapeutic effects. Chamomile contains many types of flavonoids such as apigenin and chrysoplenin, and oils that include chamazulene and bisabolol. The oil from chamomile has a light blue color. The best-known flavonoid in chamomile is apigenin (Viola 1995), which has antioxidant properties (Hertog 1993). Chamazulene has also been recently identified to have antioxidant properties (Rekka 1996).

HOW DOES CHAMOMILE WORK?

Several chemicals in chamomile, particularly apigenin, are known to influence receptors in the brain that induce relaxation and sedation (Viola 1995). These are the same receptors influenced by benzodiazepine medicines such as Valium. Therefore, chamomile theoretically would work by relaxing nerves and muscles. There are smooth muscles in the intestinal tract, around blood vessels, and many other parts of the body. Chamomile could perhaps help stomach ailments by relaxing the smooth muscles in the gastrointestinal system.

CHAMOMILE AND SLEEP

Studies on mice have shown apigenin to have sedating properties (Viola 1995). The sleep-inducing properties of chamomile are gentle compared to valerian. A weak tea of chamomile could occasionally be useful at night in infants who are teething or have colic, to help them sleep.

I have tried chamomile on several occasions and find it to have only a slight sedating property. It is too weak to induce or maintain sleep. Chamomile by itself is not effective enough for most adults who suffer from significant insomnia. It needs to be combined with other herbs or supplements for a more definitive effect.

As an experiment one morning, I took twenty chamomile capsules containing 125 milligrams of the herb standardized to about 1 percent of apigenin. I opened the capsules and made a tea from them, drinking three cups over a period of an hour, from 9 to 10 A.M. At about noon, I started feeling a little sleepy and relaxed, but the feeling wore off after a couple of hours.

HISTORICAL USES OF CHAMOMILE

Formal human research with chamomile is very limited. This herb has historically been recommended for reducing gastrointestinal spasms and colic. Some people drink chamomile tea to help settle their stomach after a full meal. Doctors have also prescribed this herb for ulcers. Chamomile is most useful in gastrointestinal disorders, such as irritable bowel syndrome, that are due to, or aggravated by, nervousness and anxiety. It can be used in infants for colic.

It has been used as a mouthwash for irritation of the mouth and gums, and externally for various skin irritations, such as rashes, cuts and scrapes, and excema.

Often chamomile tea has been recommended during the day to induce a gentle relaxation.

This herb has also been recommended for mild menstrual cramps.

Much of the information on chamomile's supposed benefits are anecdotal and therefore not proved.

HOW IS IT AVAILABLE?

The most common way to ingest chamomile is as tea. Steep the tea bag for a few minutes to allow all the compounds to diffuse in the cup and sip it about an hour or so before bed. You can also buy the flowers and use two tablespoons per cup of boiling water. Steep this for a few minutes and then strain the liquid.

Capsules containing both chamomile flowers and chamomile extract are sold in a variety of dosages:

Chamomile extract 125 milligrams, standardized to contain 1.2 percent apigenin

Chamomile flowers containing 350 milligrams, nonstandardized. This product was not an extract and the bottle did not indicate the percent of apigenin.

Chamomile flowers containing 400 milligrams, nonstandardized

You can swallow the capsules, or open them, empty the contents into a glass, and pour hot water in the glass to make a tea.

Alcoholic tinctures are available, and you can use between 1 to 5 milliliters mixed in a liquid, an hour or so before bed. You may also find dermatological preparations that include chamomile in creams, ointments, and lotions.

Chamomile is often combined with valerian, passionflower, hops, skullcap, and other herbs in a number of herbal products touted for anti-anxiety, relaxation, and sleep.

OTHER PROPERTIES OF CHAMOMILE

In one laboratory study, certain components of this herb were found to have antifungal properties (Mariann 1976).

A study in cells found extracts of chamomile to inhibit the development of poliovirus replication (Vilagines 1985). Whether components of chamomile have other antiviral properties is currently not known.

Helianol, an alcohol found in this herb, has antiinflammatory abilities (Akihisa 1996). The flavonoid apigenin also has antiinflammatory properties.

Apigenin inhibits skin tumor formation and could be useful as an addition to sunscreens (Wei 1990, Lepley 1997).

Apigenin may have anti–liver tumor properties by reversing the harmful effects of toxins with respect to the proper communication among liver cells (Chaumontet 1997).

SIDE EFFECTS

A folk remedy recommends the use of chamomile tea as an eyewash in cases of conjunctivitis (inflammation of the lining of the eyes). Certain individuals, especially those prone to allergies, may be sensitive to the components in chamomile and could have an allergic reaction to it when applied topically. This could lead to swelling of the eyelids. Pollens are the responsible allergens (Subiza 1990).

Rare cases of allergies could also occur from ingestion of chamomile tea, particularly in individuals who suffer from other allergies. A report in the *Journal of Allergy and Clinical Immunology* tells of an eight-year-old boy who had a severe, almost life-threatening reaction to chamomile tea ingestion (Subiza 1989). This patient suffered from severe hay fever and bronchial asthma caused by a variety of pollens of grass, olive, and mugwort. One of my patients who suffer from allergies reported a slight runny nose and itchy eyes the morning after drinking chamomile tea.

It is prudent for anyone who has severe allergies to plants of the daisy family, particularly ragweed, to avoid the use of chamomile.

SUMMARY

Chamomile tea is helpful as a mild relaxing agent. However, by itself, it may be too weak for those who have a moderate to strong case of nervousness or insomnia. One can certainly combine chamomile with other antianxiety or sedating herbs. For instance, you can make a cup of tea in the evening with a bag of valerian and chamomile, and even add passionflower, hops, and skullcap. Chamomile could also be useful in mild cases of stomach upset.

With the availability of chamomile extracts, it is now possible to ingest much more of the ingredients than was previously possible. We may eventually find therapeutic potentials from larger doses of chamomile extracts that were previously impractical to ingest from the tea.

Because of its content of flavonoids, such as apigenin, drinking chamomile tea on a regular basis could have some health-promoting effects. However, there are quite a number of other herbs that contain beneficial chemicals. You may want to stock a variety of teas in your kitchen and each day drink a different one. Chamomile, though, is one of the better-tasting teas.

19
SKULLCAP

Skullcap (or scullcap, *Scuttelaria lateriflora*) is a member of the mint family with blue flowers native to North America. In Europe, it is added to many nighttime herbal supplements. There are a number of species of skullcap. One of the common Asian species is known as *Scuttellaria baicalensis*.

Historically, skullcap has had a bad rap. More than fifty years ago, when skullcap was still on *The National Formulary*, the 1943 edition of the *Dispensary of the United States* declared, "Skullcap is as destitute of medicinal properties as a plant may well be, not even being aromatic. When taken internally, it produces no very obvious effects, and probably is of no medicinal value."

WHAT'S IN SKULLCAP?

Several volatile oils are present in the leaves of the herb, in addition to flavonoids such as scutellarin, wogonin, and baicalein. Most of the studies published with skullcap have been done on the Asian variety. Laboratory examination of flavonoid compounds within *Scutellaria baicalensis* have shown them to have antiviral (Nagai 1995), antiinflammatory (Huang 1994), and antithrombotic properties (Kimura 1997).

USES

Skullcap has been traditionally recommended for insomnia, stress, and premenstrual syndrome. No formal studies are available to determine this herb's effectiveness in these conditions.

HOW IS IT AVAILABLE?

Skullcap is often combined with other over-the-counter sedative herbs as sleep remedies. One or two teaspoons of the dried leaves can be steeped in hot water to make a tea. The tea can be drunk about an hour or two before bed.

Skullcap is also available as a tincture and in capsules. One company markets a skullcap product containing 340 milligrams of the herb, while another sells pills that include 450 milligrams. However, it is usually difficult to find skullcap sold by itself. In most cases it is part of a combination of herbs marketed for sleep.

SIDE EFFECTS

A 1989 report described liver damage that occurred in four women who had been ingesting high doses of skullcap on a regular basis for the relief of stress (MacGregor 1989). The occasional ingestion of skullcap has not shown to have any untoward effects.

MY PERSONAL EXPERIENCE

One evening, about an hour before bed, I opened ten capsules of skullcap, each containing 420 milligrams of the herb. I poured the contents in a glass and added hot water, then drank the tea. I went to bed at midnight, and at about 3 A.M. I awoke feeling alert and had difficulty in going back to sleep.

The next day, I poured forty drops of the tincture in a cup of soy milk and drank it at 11 A.M. By 1 P.M. I felt nothing, so I added another forty drops to a small glass of soy milk. No response. I then poured the rest of the ounce of the tincture in the soy milk and drank it over a period of half an hour. I still did not feel sleepy or sedated. Based on my limited experience with skullcap thus far, this herb's purported sedative effects have not impressed me. However, interestingly, I started feeling more alert and energetic later in the afternoon and evening. I also noticed a slight feeling of well-being. This lasted until about 11 P.M.

SUMMARY

The other herbs discussed in this book, particularly valerian and hops, are more reliable in terms of their hypnotic effect than skullcap. For anxiety, kava is the best choice. The use of skullcap by itself for sedative purposes should rarely be necessary when the other herbs are available. There should be no problems in occasionally ingesting skullcap if the herbal combination product you purchase includes this herb.

An interesting point to keep in mind is the possibility that certain flavonoids in skullcap could eventually be found to have beneficial effects in terms of antiviral, antithrombotic, and antiinflammatory effects. The clinical significance of these preliminary laboratory findings is currently not known.

CHINESE HERBS

In addition to the herbs used in Western medicine, a number of Chinese herbs have sedating or relaxing properties. According to Heiner Fruehauf, Ph.D., L.Ac., Chair of the Department of Classical Chinese Medicine at the National College of Naturopathic Medicine in Portland, Oregon, one of the best known is zizyphus. This herb can be found in some stores in the Chinatown section of many American cities. In traditional Chinese medicine, zizyphus is most often combined with other herbs that induce sedation and could be helpful in some cases of insomnia. The raw herb is ground to a powder and a teaspoon is taken directly.

HOMEOPATHIC REMEDY

Homeopathy is a system of medical treatment based on the theory of treating certain diseases with very small doses of drugs. This form of therapy is very controversial and there are many skeptics in the medical community who are not convinced of homeopathy's effectiveness. However, this form of therapy also has its believers. Jeffrey Shapiro, H.D., Ph.D., a doctor of homeopathy who practices in Los Angeles, tells me that one particular homeopathic medicine, called ignatia, often recommended for individuals who are grieving, can induce sleep when two or three tablets or pellets are dissolved under the tongue an hour or so before sleep.

20

COMBINING KAVA WITH
SUPPLEMENTS AND MEDICINES

Only a few years ago, most Americans were hardly taking any supplements except for perhaps one-a-day multivitamins and calcium. Then, in the early 1990s, more and more evidence became available that many of the antioxidants, such as vitamins C and E, beta-carotene, and the mineral selenium, were potentially beneficial. So people started taking additional antioxidant pills. In 1995, the hormone craze started, initially with melatonin followed by DHEA. Thereafter, we had a great deal of media attention focused on St. John's wort, glucosamine, ginkgo, CoQ10, and other supplements. I know many people who gobble down a couple dozen or more pills a day. With all of these pills going into our bodies, how do we know the results of their interactions?

It's very difficult to predict the long-term consequences of using various supplements in combination. Countless interactions can occur in our bodies. Nevertheless, since many people are taking a variety of supplements, by the time they come across kava, it is appropriate for me to give some guidelines on how best to combine supplements, and whether there are areas of concern that should be specified. As always, you should consult your own health care practitioner before taking or combining supplements. Please note that, in almost all cases, no studies are available to verify the appropriateness of these guidelines. These viewpoints are based on my clinical experience, knowledge of how medicines and herbs work, and interviews with users. With time, more information will be available and I can make more definitive suggestions. For the latest updates, see my website (http://www.raysahelian.com).

MULTIVITAMIN AND MINERAL PILLS

Most of these pills generally contain vitamins A, B complex, and C, and several minerals in low to moderate dosages. There should be no problems at all in combining kava with these one-a-day pills.

HERBS

There is no reason to suspect kava of having any significant interactions with saw palmetto, echinacea, goldenseal, ginger, or other herbs that do not have psychoactive compounds. I have recommended ginkgo, ginseng, and kava together to patients without problems.

See Chapter 9 on kava and depression for a discussion of kava and St. John's wort.

NUTRIENTS

Kava should not interfere with nutrients such as glucosamine, or reasonable doses of anti-oxidants such as coenzyme Q10, lipoic acid, and others. High doses of coenzyme Q10 or lipoic acid can induce overstimulation.

AMINO ACIDS

There should be no problems in using kava with small amounts of different amino acids. There are at least two amino acids that are known to increase alertness and energy, tyrosine and phenylalanine. They are sometimes used in combination with other supplements to treat depression. One problem with these amino acids is that they can, in higher dosages, lead to irritability and anxiety. Kava would potentially be able to counteract these side effects. However, an even better option is to lower the dosages of these amino acids so that they don't cause any side effects.

HORMONES

Several natural hormones are available without a prescription. These include pregnenolone (the grandmother of all the adrenal hormones), DHEA (the mother of the sex hormones), and androstenedione (son of DHEA and direct precursor to testosterone and estrogens).

As a rule, high doses of these hormones lead to irritability and aggressiveness, along with inducing anxiety. Low to moderate doses of these hormones actually reduce anxiety and even provide a sense of well-being. I consider any dosage above 10 milligrams a high dose. Many people are misusing these hormones by taking dosages beyond the physiological requirements of the body.

If you feel anxious while taking these hormones, kava is a good option to try. However, my suggestion is to take a lower dosage of the hormones and thus avoid the side effects of irritability and nervousness in the first place. However, if you are prescribed high dosages of these hormones for a particular medical condition, and you need temporary help to combat the anxiety, the use of kava is justified. Of course, the regular use of hormones should be done only under the supervision of a health care professional.

Many postmenopausal women are on estrogen replacement therapy. There are no known contraindications for using kava in conjunction with estrogens.

SLEEP SUPPLEMENTS

Valerian is a fernlike plant whose root has compounds, such as valerenic acid and valeprotriates, that influence GABA receptors in the brain, leading to relaxation and sleep. The usual dose for sleep is about 300 to 400 milligrams. When combined with kava, the dose should be reduced by half. For instance, kava can be taken at 40 milligrams, valerian at 100 to 200 milligrams. If you are particularly sensitive to medicines, initially use a smaller amount of these herbs.

Hops, passionflower, skullcap, and chamomile are other herbs you may find combined with kava. As always, to be on the cautious side, initially take half a capsule an hour before bed to see how you tolerate these herbs, or half the recommended dosage on the bottle. Many herbal supplements available in stores use the combination of several herbs known for their relaxing or sedative effects. These are generally safe to take, and no significant side effects have been reported in the medical literature.

As to melatonin, it is best not to exceed a dose of 1 milligram when you combine it with other sedative herbs. Otherwise, you may feel groggy in the morning.

SEDATIVES

Until testing is done with the combination of kava and various sedative drugs, it is best not to combine them unless you are guided by an experienced physician familiar with both pharmaceutical drugs and herbal therapy.

A 1996 letter to the editor of the *Annals of Internal Medicine*, titled "Coma from the health food store," reads, "A 54-year-old man was hospitalized at our center in a lethargic and disoriented state. His medications included alprazolam [Xanax], cimetidine [Tagamet], and terazosin [Hytrin]. His vital signs and results of laboratory studies were normal. His alcohol level was negative, and a drug screen was positive for benzodiazepines. He became more alert after several hours and stated that he had been taking a 'natural tranquilizer' called kava for the past 3 days, bought from a local health food store. He denied overdosing on the kava or alprazolam" (Almeida, 1996).

In my opinion, there seems to be a bias here in terms of the sensational title of this letter. Why isn't it called "Coma from the pharmacy"? The drug alprazolam is much more likely to induce coma than is kava. It's also possible that the combination of alprazolam with the other two drugs caused the problem.

It's important to keep in mind that kava has some actions on the nervous system, such as an influence on GABA receptors, that are similar to benzodiazepines (such as Xanax). In the case of this lethargic gentleman, the problem was more likely due to Xanax since it is more sedating than kava.

Having reported the above, I cannot rule out the possibility that some individuals could benefit from the combination of low doses of benzodiazepines, or other antianxiety drugs, and kava. For instance, if kava alone is not sufficient in reducing anxiety, it may be combined with a low dose of pharmaceutical medicines such as buspirone and benzodiazepines.

These combinations have not been tested and, therefore, one would need to be guided by a physician.

CAN I SWITCH FROM SEDATIVES TO KAVA?

Let's assume you've been on a sedative or tranquilizer, like Xanax, three times a day for a month or less. It is best while you make the transition that over a period of a week you reduce the dose to twice a day, then once a day. The day you go off the Xanax, you can start kava once a day. If you tolerate it well, the next day you can increase the dose to twice a day, and the following day to three times a day.

Of course, if you've been on a sedative for many months or years, the transition process has to be very slow. This could take a month or two, or even more.

ANTIDEPRESSANTS

A common question I am asked during radio interviews or while giving lectures on supplements is whether kava can be used in combination with traditional antidepressants. No studies have yet been published addressing this subject. Therefore, our knowledge in this area is very limited and we only have anecdotes to rely on.

Currently used antidepressants include selective serotonin reuptake inhibitors (SSRIs) such as Paxil, Zoloft, and Prozac, or tricyclic antidepressants such as Elavil. In high dosages, some of the SSRIs cause agitation and anxiety. Hence, kava, due to its relaxing properties, could theoretically take the edge off. This is all uncharted territory, and whenever we travel into these grounds, we should be extremely cautious. This means that if you plan to use kava with antidepressants, the initial dosages of kava added to the existing medicines should be very low. A starting kavalactone dosage of 30 to 50 milligrams is one option. It is also wise to decrease the dosage of the particular medicine on the day of adding the kava.

It's quite possible that some patients may benefit from the combination of kava with other medicines used in psychiatry. Andrew, a thirty-seven-year-old software engineer, reports, "I have been in treatment for depression, generalized anxiety disorder, and obsessive-compulsive disorder for several years. I have taken a number of antidepressants, Paxil being the latest, and I have taken kava extracts fairly often throughout this time.

I find kava to be calming, relaxing, and mildly euphoric. I have never had any problems or side effects with kava."

KAVA AND CAFFEINE

Many people drink coffee to wake up and be alert. However, caffeine can sometimes lead to irritability and anxiety. The relaxing and anti-anxiety effects of kava could be helpful in cases of the caffeine jitters. However, it's best not to make it a habit of combining the two, since studies have not been done with this combination.

21

SUMMARY AND PRACTICAL
RECOMMENDATIONS

If you currently have a mild or moderate case of anxiety, and you need temporary help, kava may provide you with benefits (assuming, of course, that you've tried nonpill approaches without success). Kava is a good alternative to benzodiazepines and tranquilizer drugs currently prescribed for anxiety. If you have a persistent case of anxiety, and kava is not effective, then you may have to resort temporarily to prescription medicines—with the supervision of your health care practitioner.

- Start with one kava capsule of 40 to 80 milligrams of kavalactones in the evening for two days. If this is effective, then you can stay on this dose.

- If this evening dose is not effective by itself, then you can take a second dose during the day. Continue on this twice a day, dosing for another two days.
- If you still feel tense and anxious, you can add a third dose, and you can spread these three doses throughout the day.
- If you're still not feeling any effects, you can temporarily increase your dosage to between 100 to 200 milligrams of kavalactones.
- Once you are better, you can reduce your dosage and eventually go off the kava. If, with time, your symptoms return, you can start kava again.

Please remember that kava is not meant to be consumed for more than six months. As with any medicine, it should be used as needed and then discontinued.

FOR SLEEP

Of all the herbs discussed in this book, valerian is the most consistent as to its sleep-inducing effects, followed by hops. Passionflower and chamomile are weak, and skullcap is very inconsistent. Kava more often produces alertness rather than sleepiness and thus should not be relied on as a sleep-inducing agent to be taken shortly before bed. However, some individuals find that the relaxing effects of kava help them sleep better. Kava could provide a deeper sleep if taken several hours before bed, allowing time for the alertness to wear off.

The herbal renaissance in North America has started, and more people are realizing the potential of herbs and supplements to play a positive role in medicine. There is no doubt that kava, valerian, and other herbs will become more popular with time. For the latest information and recommendations, see my regularly updated website (http://www.raysahelian.com).

22

PERSONAL STORIES

Having recommended kava to dozens of patients, interviewed more than a hundred users of kava and other herbs, and having discussed its properties with researchers and physicians, it has became apparent to me that the response to kava ingestion is not consistent. The following are a sampling of these responses.

I have been under a lot of stress lately. Each morning I take two kava capsules and find that this herb helps me relax. I have had migraine headaches and feverfew helps me deal with the migraine. I haven't found any untoward reaction mixing the feverfew and the kava. For many years I've had a knee injury. Kava is able to slightly ease the pain. Although valerian helps me sleep at night, I have not found it to be very effective during the day for anxiety. I take valerian at night combined with passionflower and lavender.—VC, thirty, Orlando, Florida

I took three kava pills of 150 milligrams (30 percent kavalactones) each at 7 P.M. An hour later, I had not noticed any effects, so I took two more pills. A half hour later I took another two pills, for a total of seven pills of 45 milligrams of kavalactones each, equaling 315 milligrams. At about 9:30 P.M. I noticed a calming effect with a mild euphoria. I happened to be having dinner with a few friends in a Thai restaurant. The company was very pleasant and I had a good time. I didn't sleep well overnight. I think the kava may have interfered with my sleep.— RD, twenty-five, Burbank, California

A small amount of kava, such as 50 to 70 milligrams of kavalactones, helps me relax and sleep, but when I take too high a dose it actually causes me to be alert.—DG, fifty-five, Hollywood, Florida

I've tried a lot of kava products, and none of the capsules or tablets do a thing for me.

What seems to be effective are the liquid extracts. A few full drops under the tongue, and you can feel the kava within a couple of minutes—calming, relaxing, a marvelous herb!—JU, forty-four, New York City

I've tried the liquid extract. The taste is horrible. I had a few of my friends try it too, with the same response—horrible taste and it didn't do a thing for me. You must have to take a lot of the liquid extract to feel something.—KI, thirty-two, Chicago

My Chinese doctor gave me a combination of kava and American ginseng about ten days ago. It took about a week but I am starting to realize that I have less anxiety and do not need that small amount of Xanax to get me going. In fact I feel mellow. So far it has helped me more than a lot of other medications.—AA, thirty, Jacksonville, Florida

There's been a lot of stress in my life lately and I've been nervous and unhappy. My girlfriend left me for someone else. I can't stop thinking about her. I don't want to take any prescription drugs and a friend told me about kava. I recorded my experience with this herb.

Day one: I dissolved half a teaspoon of a concentrated kava powder in water and drank it as I would a regular glass of water. The taste was intolerable. Five minutes into it I felt relaxed, but content. I could lie on the beach (maybe somewhere in the South Pacific) and not wonder about what is happening anywhere else in the world. Sort of in my own little world. I also noticed visual enhancement. Objects looked three-dimensional. I noticed the contrast in colors of the telephone and monitor, black and gray respectively—they complemented each other, sort of like a belt and shoes. Looking over to my side I saw a coworker's red sweater to be much brighter than usual. It's been about ten minutes now and I noticed a slight headache and nausea. I think the dose I took was too high.

Day two: Last night I slept for a total of nine hours, which is unusual for me. I regularly sleep six hours. Today I am trying a quarter teaspoon of the same powder but this time in soy milk instead of water and drinking it over a period of fifteen minutes. The taste is definitely more tolerable. The headache hit once again about ten minutes after I drank my concoction. It's been about two hours now and I am feeling good, at ease. I am taking things more lightly, not so concerned about my recent heartbreaking love life. For the first time in many weeks I actually feel happy.

In the evening I was very creative, my thoughts were extremely clear. It was amazing. My friend called while I was working on my personal Web site and I immediately got off the phone because I was afraid I would lose my sudden burst of creativity. My mind was functioning more efficiently than usual.

Day three: Today I took four pills of 70 milligrams of kavalactones each. I did not feel the same effects as I did on day one. No visual enhancement such as brighter colors or three-dimensional effects that I experienced on the half-teaspoon dose I took the first day. I do not even feel the relaxed state that I did yesterday. Maybe it was the higher concentration of kavalactones in the previous brand. It was supposed to be a more potent formula. It's been about three hours now. I feel tired and sleepy, not to the point where I have to take a nap but I'm not completely alert either. I am also not very focused in what I have just been reading this past half hour. I took two more pills. Ten minutes later I felt more alert. I find that initially, after taking kava, I am more alert. Then about three hours later I feel sleepy.

Day four: I took two capsules today and didn't notice much. About three hours later I took an additional two capsules and felt a subtle enhancement in mood. My coworkers noticed that I was being more talkative and cheerful. They mentioned that I was acting happier than they had seen me for weeks. The feeling lasted a few hours.

Day five: After almost two hours of bumper-to-bumper traffic on the way to work this morning, I needed kava. It took two capsules and I'm feeling much better, more relaxed, cheerier.

I find that kava, although its effects are not always clearly noticeable, has been helpful in the past few days in dealing with some of the stress in my life.—JM, twenty-eight, Brentwood, California

I currently use a blend of kava, hops, and valerian root in a gel capsule. This has no taste (although I can taste it if I burp after taking it) and relaxes me, almost puts me to sleep. In the past I have had kava as a tincture, which tasted absolutely terrible. I became very close to throwing up. It coated my tongue and throat very noticeably. I had little in the way of effects, as I was concentrating with my lunch. I don't like the taste of kava, and for this reason I prefer capsules. However, I'm not sure that I have ever had the "true" kava experience. The capsules I take contain other herbs that also induce relaxation and I cannot determine which particular effects are due to which herb.—LK, Denver

RESOURCES

You can see posts about kava on various news-groups including misc.health.alternative; rec.drugs.smart; alt.folklore.herbs; alt.support.anxiety; alt.drugs; and sci.med.nutrition. Additionally, you can do a search for kava on the search engine dejanews, or see websites pertaining to kava through Webcrawler or Altavista. See the last page to subscribe to *Longevity Research Update*.

FOR MORE INFORMATION

Herb Research Foundation
Rob McCaleb, president
1007 Pearl Street
Suite 200
Boulder, CO 80302
303-449-2265
www.herbs.org
info@herbs.org

RESOURCES

American Botanical Council
Marc Blumenthal, executive director
PO Box 201660
Austin, TX 78720
512-331-8868
abc@herbalgram.org
The ABC publishes an excellent quarterly journal called *Herbalgram*. Issue 39 of the journal included a special report updating Dr. Yadhu Singh's 1992 review article on the history of kava.

Herbs For Health
Logan Chamberlain, publisher
201 East Fourth Street
Loveland, CO 80537
970-669-7672
www.interweave.com
Bimonthly magazines on herbs

BOOKS

Kava: Castleman, Michael. *The Healing Herbs*. Bantam Books, 1991. Includes a good description of dozens of herbs.
Lebot, Vincent, Mark Merlin, and Lamont Lindstrom. *The Pacific Elixir*. Healing Arts Press, 1997. Includes research on the botany, chemistry, ethnobotany, pharmacology, social usage, distribution, and economic potential.
Valerian: Hobbs, Christopher. *The Relaxing and Sleep Herb*. Capitola, California: Botanica Press, 1993. A good review of valerian.
Tyler, Varro. *The Honest Herbal*. Binghamton, New York: Pharmaceutical Products Press, 1993. Brown, Donald. *Herbal Prescriptions for Better Health*. Rocklin, California: Prima Publishing, 1995.

REFERENCES

KAVA

Almeida, J. C., and E. W. Grimsley. 1996. Coma from the health food store: Interaction between kava and alprazolam. *Ann. Int. Med.* 125:940–41. Letter to the editor from two doctors at the Memorial Medical Center in Savannah, Georgia.

Banazak, D. 1997. Anxiety disorders in elderly patients. *J. American Board Family Practice* 10 (4):280–89.

Benton, D., J. Haller, and J. Fordy. 1995. Vitamin supplementation for 1 year improves mood. *Neuropsychobiology* 32:98–105.

Borsche, W., and B. K. Blount. 1933. Untersuchungen uber die bestandteile der kawawurzel. *Chemische Berichte* 66: 803–06.

Cantor, C. 1997. Kava and alcohol. *Medical Journal of Australia* 167:560. Letter to the editor.

Cawte, J. 1985. Psychoactive substances of the South Seas: betel, kava, and pituri. *Asut NZ J. Psychiatry* 19:83–87.

Decloitre, P. 1995. *Pacific Islands Monthly*, April, p. 44.

REFERENCES

Duffield, A. M., D. D. Jamieson, R. O. Lidgard, et al. 1989. Identification of some human urinary metabolites of the intoxicating beverage kava. *J. Chromatogr.* 475:273–81.

Duffield, P. H., and D. Jamieson. 1991. Development of tolerance to kava in mice. *Clin. Exp. Pharmacol. Physiol.* 18:571–78.

Finau, S. A., J. M. Stanhope, and I. A. Prior. 1982. Kava, alcohol, and tobacco consumption among Tongans with urbanization. *Soc. Sci. Med.* 16:35–41.

Foster, F., ed. 1897. *Reference book of practical therapeutics*. D. Appleton and Company.

Garner, L. F., and J. D. Klinger. 1985. Some visual effects caused by the beverage kava. *J. Ethnopharmacol.* 13 (3): 307–11.

Gleitz, J., A. Beile, P. Wilkens, A. Ameri, and T. Peters. 1997. Antithrombotic action of the kava pyrone kavain prepared from *Piper methysticum* on human platelets. *Planta Medica* 63:27–30. Exogenously applied arachidonic acid induced a 90 percent aggregation of platelets and the release of thromboxane A2 (TXA2) and prostaglandin E2 (PGE2). An application of kavain five minutes before AA, dose-dependently diminished aggregation and the synthesis of TXA2 and PGE2. This suggests an inhibition of cyclooxygenase.

Gleitz, J., J. Friese, A. Beile, A. Ameri, and T. Peters. 1996. Anticonvulsive action of kavain estimated from its properties on stimulated synaptosomes and sodium channel receptor sites. *Eur. J. Pharmacol.* 315:89–97. The data suggest an interaction of kavain with voltage-dependent sodium and calcium channels, thereby suppressing 4-animopyridine-induced increase in sodium and calcium and the release of endogenous glutamate.

Groth-Marnat, G., S. Leslie, and M. Renneker. 1996. Tobacco control in a traditional Fijian village: Indigenous methods of smoking cessation and relapse prevention. *Soc. Sci. Med.* 43: 473–77.

Haberlein, J., G. Boonen, and M. A. Beck. 1997. *Piper methysticum*: Enantiomeric separation of kavapyrones by high performance liquid chromatography. *Planta Medica* 63:63–65.

REFERENCES

Hansel, R. 1968. Characterization and physiological activity of some kava constituents. *Pacific Science* 22:293–313.

Harrison, T. 1937. *Savage civilization*. New York: Alfred A. Knopf.

Heinze, H. J., T. F. Munte, J. Steitz, and M. Matzke. 1994. Pharmacopsychological effects of oxazepam and kava extract in a visual search paradigm assessed with event-related potentials. *Pharmacopsychiatry* 27:224–30.

Herberg, K. W. 1993. Effect of special extract WS 1490 combined with ethyl alcohol on safety-relevant performance parameters. *Blutalkohol* 30:96–105.

Hocart, C. H., B. Fankhauser, and D. W. Buckle. 1993. Chemical archaeology of kava, a potent brew. *Rapid Commun. Mass Specrom.* 7:219–24.

Hocking, L. B., and H. G. Koenig. 1995. Anxiety in medically ill older patients: A review and update. *Int. J. Psychiatry Med.* 25:221–38.

Holm, E., U. Staedt, J. Heep, C. Kortsik, F. Behne, A. Kaske, and I. Mennicke. 1991. The action profile of D, L-kavain: Cerebral sites and sleep-wakefulness-rhythm in animals. *Arzneimiielforschung* 41 (7):673–83. Cats were injected with intraperitoneal kavain and monitored with EEG, electromyograms, and subcortical evoked potentials. It was concluded from the findings that limbic structures and, in particular, the amygdalar complex represent the preferential sites of action for both kavain and the kava extract. The participation of these structures in modulating emotional processes may explain the promotion of sleep, even in the absence of sedation. There is no congruity of kavain with either the tricyclic thymoleptics or the benzodiazepines regarding the profile of neurophysiological effects.

Jamieson, D. D., and P. H. Duffield. 1990a. The antinociceptive actions of kava components in mice. *Clin. Exp. Pharmacol. Physiol.* 17:495–507.

———. 1990b. Positive interaction of ethanol and kava resin in mice. *Clin. Exp. Pharmacol. Physiol.* 17:509–14.

Jamieson, D. D., P. H. Duffield, D. Cheng, and A. M. Duffield. 1989. Comparison of the central nervous system activity of the aqueous and lipid extract of kava. *Arch. Int. Pharmacodyn Ther.* 301 (Animal): 66–80.

REFERENCES

Jappe, U., I. Franke, D. Reinhold, and H. P. Gollnick. 1998. Sebotropic drug reaction resulting from kava-kava extract therapy: A new entity? *J. Am. Acad. Dermatol.* 38 (1):104–06.

Jussofie, A., A. Schmiz, and C. Hiemke. 1994. Kavapyrone enriched extract from *Piper methysticum* as modulator of the GABA-binding site in different regions of rat brain. *Psychopharmacology* 116:469–74. "Our findings suggest that one way kavapyrones might mediate sedative effects in vivo is through effects on GABA-A receptor binding."

Keledjian, J., P. Duffield, D. Jamieson, R. Lidgard, and A. Duffield. 1988. Uptake into mouse brain of four compounds present in the psychoactive beverage kava *J. Pharm. Sci.* 77 (12):1003–06.

Kinzler, E., J. Kromer, and E. Lehmann. 1991. Effect of a special kava extract in patients with anxiety, tension, and excitation states of non-psychotic genesis: Double-blind study with placebos over 4 weeks. *Arzneimittelforschung* 41:584–88.

Laux, G. 1997. Pharmacotherapy. *Ther Umsch* 54 (10):595–99.

Lehmann, D., E. Kinzler, and J. Friedemann, 1996. Efficacy of a special kava extract (*Piper methysticum*) in patients with states of anxiety, tension and excitedness of nonmental origin—A double-blind placebo-controlled study of four weeks treatment. *Phytomedicine* 3:113–19.

Lemert, E. M. 1976. Koni, kona, kava, orange-beer culture of the Cook Islands. *J. Stud. Alcohol* 37:565–85.

Magura, E., M. Kopanista, J. Gleitz, T. Peters, and O. Krishtal. 1997. Kava extract ingredients, (+)-methysticin and (+/−)-kavain inhibit voltage-operated Na(+)-channels in rat CA1 hippocampal neurons. *Neuroscience* 81 (2):345–51.

Mathews, J. D., M. D. Riley, et al. 1988. Effects of the heavy usage of kava on physical health: Summary of a pilot survey in an aboriginal community. *Med. J. Aust.* 148: 548–55.

Munte, T. F., H. J. Heinze, M. Matzke, and J. Steitz. 1993. Effects of oxazepam and an extract of kava roots (*Piper methysticum*) on event-related potentials in a word recognition task. *Neuropsychology* 27:46–53.

REFERENCES

Norton, S. A., and P. Ruze. 1994. Kava dermopathy. *J. Am. Acad. Dermatol.* 31:89–97. The history of kava dermopathy from Captain Cook's early reports to its presence today.

Rasmussen, A. K., R. R. Scheline, E. Solheim, and R. Hansel. 1979. Metabolism of some kava pyrones in the rat. *Xenobiotica* 9:1–16.

Ruze, P. 1990. Kava-induced dermopathy: A niacin deficiency? *Lancet* 335:1442–45.

St. Claire, D. 1997. *The Herbal medicine cabinet: Preparing natural remedies at home.* Berkeley: Celestial Arts Publishers. A how-to guide for preparing tinctures, ointment, teas, and extracts in your own kitchen.

Schelosky, L., C. Raffauf, et al. 1995. Kava and dopamine antagonism. *J. Neurol. Neurosurg. Psychiatry* 45 (5): 639–40. Letter to the editor. Four case histories are presented, which indicate that the sedative effects of kava might result from dopamine antagonistic properties. "This possibility is also supported by clinical findings of beneficial effects of kava on schizophrenic symptoms in Australian Aborigines (Cawte, 1985). Experimentally, kava extracts have been shown to antagonize sterotypies induced by apomorphine in mice. We draw attention to the potential of extrapyramidal side effects of kava preparations and caution their use, particularly in elderly patients."

Seitz, U., A. Ameri, H. Pelzer, J. Gleitz, and T. Peters. 1997. Relaxation of evoked contractile activity of isolated guinea-pig ileum by (+/−)-kavain. *Planta Medica* 63 (4): 303–06. Kavain dose-dependently reduced contractions of ileum evoked by carbachol. "The kava pyrone kavain acts in a non-specific musculotropic way on the smooth muscle membrane of the ileum."

Seitz, U., A. Schule, and J. Gleitz. 1997. [3H]-monoamine uptake inhibition properties of kava pyrones. *Planta Medica* 63 (6):548–49.

Singh, Y. N. 1983. Effects of kava on neuromuscular transmission and muscle contractility. *J. Ethnopharmacol.* 7 (3):267–76.

REFERENCES

———. 1992. Kava: An overview. *J. Ethnopharmacol.* 37: 13–45. Great review article.

Shulgin, A. T. 1973. The narcotic pepper: The chemistry and pharmacology of *Piper methysticum* and related species. *Bulletin on Narcotics* 59–74.

Spillane, P., D. Fisher, and B. Currie. 1997. Neurological manifestations of kava intoxication. *Medical Journal of Australia*, August 4.

Suss, R., and P. Lehmann. 1996. Hematogenous contact eczema caused by phytogenic exemplified by kava root extract. *Hauzarzt* 47:459–61.

Volz, H. P., and M. Kieser. 1997. Kava-kava extract WS 1490 versus placebo in anxiety disorders—A randomized placebo-controlled 25-week outpatient trial. *Pharmacopsychiat.* 30:1–5.

Walden, J. J. von Wegerer, U. Winter, M. Berger, and H. Grunze. 1997. Effects of kawain and dihydromethysticin on field potential changes in the hippocampus. *Neuropsychopharmacol. Biol. Psychiatry* 21 (4):697–706.

Warnecke, G. 1991. Psychosomatic dysfunctions in the female climacteric: Clinical effectiveness and tolerance of kava extract WS 1490. *Fortschr. Med.* 109:119–22. "The course of parameters as depressive mood (DSI), subjective well-being (patient diary), severity of the disease (CGI), and the climacteric symptomatology (Kuppermann Index and Schneider scale) over the overall period of treatment demonstrate a high level of efficacy of kava extract WS 1490 in neurovegetative and psychosomatic dysfunctions in the climacteric, associated with very good tolerance of the preparation."

Xian-guo, H., L. Long-ze, and L. Li-zhi. 1997. Electrospray high performance liquid chromotography-mass spectrometry in phytochemical analysis of kava (*piper methysticum*) extract. *Planta Medica* 63:70–74. An HPLC of the chloroform extract of kava root found thirteen kavalactones and flavokavains.

REFERENCES

VALERIAN

Andreatini, R., and J. Leite. 1994. Effect of valepotriates on the behavior of rats in the elevated plus maze during diazepam withdrawal. *Eur. J. Pharm.* 260:233–35.

Balderer, G., and A. A. Borberly. 1985. Effect of valerian on human sleep. *Psychopharmacology* (Berl) 87 (4):406–09.

Cavadas, C., I. Araujo, M. D. Cotrim, T. Anaral, et al. 1995. In vitro study on the interaction of *Valerian officinalis L.* extracts and their amino acids on GABAA receptor in rat brain. *Arzeimittelforschung* 45 (7):753–55.

Dagan, Y., N. Zisapel, D. Nof, M. Laudon, and J. Atsmon. 1997. Rapid reversal of tolerance to benzodiazepine hypnotics by treatment with oral melatonin: A case report. *Eur. Neuropsychopharmacol.* 7:157–60.

Dunaev, V., S. Trzhetsinskii, et al. 1987. Biological activity of the sum of the valepotriates isolated from *Valerian alliariifolia. Farmakol Todsikol* 50 (6):33–37.

Gerhard, U., N. Linnenbrink, C. Geroghiadou, and V. Hobi. 1996. Vigilance-decreasing effects of 2 plant-derived sedatives. *Schwiz. Rundsch. Med. Prax.* 9, 85, (15):473–81.

Hazelhoff, B., M. Malingre, et al. 1982. Antispasmodic effects of valeriana compounds: An in-vivo and in-vitro study on the guinea-pig ileum. *Arch. Int. Pharm.* 257: 274–87.

Holzl, J., and P. Godau. 1989. Receptor binding studies with *Valeriana officinalis* on the benzodiazepine receptor. *Planta Medica* 55:642.

Houghton, P. J. 1988. The biological activity of valerian and related plants. *J. Ethnopharmacol.* "Isovaleric acid is the compound which causes the odor of valerian." Great review article.

Kohnen, R., and W. D. Oswald. 1988. The effects of valerian, propranolol, and their combination on activation, performance, and mood of healthy volunteers under social stress conditions. *Pharmacopsychiatry* 21 (6):447–48. "The two drugs act independently of each other."

Leathwood, P., and F. Chauffard. 1983. Quantifying the effects of mild sedatives. *J. Psychiat. Res.* 17 (2):115–22.

———. 1985. Aqueous extract of valerian reduces latency to fall asleep in man. *Planta Medica* 2:144–48.

Leathwood, P. D., F. Chauffard, E. Heck, and R. Munoz-Box. 1982. Aqueous extract of valerian root *(Valeriana officinalis L.)* improves sleep quality in man. *Pharmacol. Biochem. Behav.* 17 (1):65–71.

Leuschner, J., J. Muller, and M. Rudman. 1993. Characterization of the central nervous depressant activity of a commercially available valerian root extract. *Arzneimittelforschung* 43 (6):638–41.

Lindahl, O., and L. Lindwall. 1989. Double blind study of a valerian preparation. *Pharm. Biochem. Behav.* 32 (4): 1065–66.

Mennini, T., P. Bernasconi, E. Bombardelli, et al. 1993. In vitro study on the interaction of extracts and pure compounds from *Valeriana officinalis* roots with GABA, benzodiazepine and barbiturate receptors in rat brain. *Fitoterapia* 64:291–300.

Santos, M. S., F. Ferreira, A. P. Cunha, A. P. Carvalho, et al. 1994. An aqueous extract of valerian influences the transport of GABA in synaptosomes. *Planta Medica* 60 (3): 278–79. Very high doses of valepotriates administered intraperitoneally induced some retarded ossification in the offspring. This did not occur when valepotriates were given orally.

Schulz, H., C. Stolz, and J. Muller. 1994. The effect of valerian extract on sleep polygraphy in poor sleepers: A pilot study. *Pharmacopsychiatry* 27 (4):147–51.

Tufik, S., K. Fujita, M. de L. Seabra, and L. L. Lobo. 1994. Effects of a prolonged administration of valepotriates in rats on the mothers and their offspring. *J. Ethnopharmacol.* 41 (1–2):39–44.

REFERENCES

Veith, J., and G. Schneider. 1986. The influence of some degradation products of valpotriates on the motor activity in mice. *Planta Medica* 179–83.

Willey, L. B., S. Mady, D. Cobaugh, and P. Wax. 1995. Valerian overdose: A case report. *Vet. Human Toxicol.* 37 (4):364–65.

Wolman, R. S. 1972. Some important abuses practiced upon the valerian. *Clin. Ped.* 11:655–57.

HOPS

Haas, L. F. 1995. Neurological stamp: *Humulus lupulus. J. Neurol. Neurosurg. Psychiatry* 58 (2):152.

Langezaal, C. R., A. Chandra, and J. J. Scheffer. 1992. Antimicrobial screening of essential oils and extracts of some *Humulus lupulus L.* cultivars. *Pharm. Weekbl. Sci.* 11, 14 (6):353–56.

Simpson, W. J., and A. R. Smith. 1992. Factors affecting antibacterial activity of hop compounds and their derivatives. *J. Appl. Bacteriol.* 72 (4):327–34.

Tobe, H., M. Kubota, M. Yamguchi, T. Kocha, and T. Aoyagi. 1997. Apoptosis to HL-60 by humulone. *Biosci. Biotechnol. Biochem* 61 (6):1027–29.

Tobe, H., Y. Muraki, K. Kitamura, et al. 1997. Bone resorption inhibitors from hop extract. *Biosci. Biotechnol. Biochem.* 61 (1):158–59.

Verschuere, M., P. Sandra, and F. David. 1992. Fractionation by SFE and microcolumn analysis of the essential oil and the bitter principles of hops. *J. Chromatogr. Sci.* 30 (10):388–91.

Yasukawa, K., M. Takeuchi, and M. Takido. 1995. Humulon, a bitter in the hop, inhibits tumor promotion by 12-O-tetradecanoylphorbol-13-acetate in two-stage carcinogenesis in mouse skin. *Oncology* 52 (2):156–58.

REFERENCES

PASSIONFLOWER

Brasseur, T., and L. Angenot. 1984. *Journal de Pharmacologie Belge*. 39(1), 15.

Lohdelink, J., and H. Kating. 1974. Zur Frage des Vorkommens von Harmanalkaloiden in Passiflora-arten. *Planta Medica* 25:101–04.

Lutomski, J., and F. Wrocinski. 1960. Pharmacodynamic properties of *Passiflora incarnata* preparations: The effect of alkaloid and flavonoid components on pharmacodynamic properties of the raw materials. *Bialetyn Instytut Roslin Leczniczych* 6:176–94.

Quercia, V. 1978. Identification and determination of vitexin and isovitexin in *Passiflora incarnata* extracts. *J. Chromatog*. 161:396–402.

Rahman, K., L. Krenn B. Kopp, M. Schubert-Zsilavecz, K. K. Mayer, and W. Kuberka. 1997. Isoscoparin-2-0-glucoside from *passiflora incarnata*. *Phytochemistry* 45:1093–94.

Solbakken, A., G. Rorbakken, and T. Gundersen. 1997. Nature medicine as intoxicant. *Tidsskr Nor Laegeforen* 20, 117 (8):1140–41. Five patients were admitted to a hospital with altered consciousness after taking Relaxir, a remedy for insomnia and restlessness, produced mainly from the fruit of the passionflower.

Soulimani, R., C. Younos, S. Jarmouni, D. Bousta, R. Misslin, and F. Mortier. 1997. Behavioral effects of *Passiflora incarnata L.* and its indole alkaloid and flavonoid derivatives and maltol in the mouse. *J. Ethnopharmacology* 57:11–20.

Speroni, E., and A. Minghetti. 1988. Neuropharmacological activity of extracts from *passiflora incarnate*. *Planta Medica* 17:488–91.

Wolfman, C., H. Viola, Paladini, et al. 1994. Possible anxiolytic effects of chrysin, a central benzodiazepine receptor ligand isolated from *Passiflora coerulea*. *Pharm. Biochem. Beh.* 47:1–4. Chrysin, a flavone, is one of the major components with influence of benzodiazepine receptor.

REFERENCES

CHAMOMILE

Akihisa, T., K. Yasukawa, H. Oinuma, and Y. Kasahara. 1996. Triterpene alcohols from the flowers of compositae and their anti-inflammatory effects. *Phytochemistry* 43 (6):1255–60. Helionol was the predominant component in the triterpene alcohol fractions in chamomile. The triterpene alcohols showed anti-inflammatory activity.

Chaumontet, C., C. Droumaguet, V. Bex, C. Heberden, et al. 1997. Flavonoids (apigenin, tangeretin) counteract tumor promoter-induced inhibition of intercellular communication of rat liver epithelial cells. *Cancer Lett.* 19, 114 (1–2):207–10.

Hertog, M. G., E. J. Feskens, P. C. Hollman, M. B. Katan, et al. 1993. Dietary antioxidant flavonoids and risk of coronary heart disease: The Zutphen Elderly Study. *Lancet* 23, 342 (8878):1007–11.

Lepley, D. M., and J. C. Pelling. 1997. Induction of p21/WAF1 and G1 cell-cycle arrest by the chemopreventive agent apigenin. *Mol. Carcinog.* 19 (2):74–82. Laboratory studies with apigenin were done on fibroblasts. "Apigenin treatment produced a G1 cell-cycle arrest by inhibiting cdk2 kinase activity and the phophorylation of Rb and inducing the cdk inhibitor p21/WAF1, all of which may mediate its chemopreventive activities in vivo. To our knowledge this is the first report of a chemopreventive agent inducing p21/WAF1, a known downstream effector of the p53 tumor suppressor protein."

Mariann, S., V. P. Gizella, and F. Ede. 1976. Antifungal effect of the biologically active components of *Matricaria chamomilla*. *Acta Pharm. Hung.* 46 (5–6):232–47.

Merfort, I., J. Heilmann, U. Hagedorn-Leweke, and B. C. Lippold. 1994. In vivo skin penetration studies of camomile flavones. *Pharmazie* 49 (7):509–11. Camomile flavones apigenin and luteolin were able to penetrate skin and reach into deeper skin layers. "This is important for their topical use as antiphlogistic [anti-inflammatory] agents."

Rekka, E. A., A. P. Kourounakis, and P. N. Kourounakis. 1996. Investigation of the effect of chamazulene on lipid peroxidation and free radical processes. Res. Commun. *Mol. Pathol. Pharmacol.* 92 (3):361–64.

Subiza, J., J. L. Subiza, M. Alonso, M. Hinojosa, et al. 1990. Allergic conjunctivitis to chamomile tea. *Ann. Allergy* 65 (2):127–32.

Subiza, J., J. L. Subiza, M. Hinojosa, R. Garcia, et al. 1989. Anaphylactic reaction after the ingestion of chamomile tea: A study of cross-reactivity with other composite pollens. *J. Allergy Clin. Immunol.* 84 (3):353–58.

Vilagines, P., P. Delaveau, and R. Vilagines. 1985. Inhibition of poliovirus replication by an extract of *Matricaria chamomilla. C R Acad. Sci. III* 301 (6):289–94.

Viola, H., C. Wasowski, M. Levi de Stein, C. Wolfman, et al. 1995. Apigenin, a component of *Matricaria recutita* flowers, is a central benzodiazepine receptors-ligand with anxiolytic effects. *Planta Medica* 61 (3):213–16. Apigenin is identified as 5,7,4-trihydroxyflavone. It competitively inhibited the binding of flunitrazepam but had no effect on muscarinic receptors, alpha 1-adrenoceptors, and the binding of muscimol to GABAA receptors. No anticonvulsant action was detected. Apigenin had sedative effects in mice only in very high dosages.

Wei, H., L. Tye, E. Bresnick, and D. F. Birt. 1990. Inhibitory effect of apigenin, a plant flavonoid, on epidermal ornithine decarboxylase and skin tumor promotion in mice. *Cancer Res.* 1, 50 (3):499–502. Topical application of apigenin on skin tumorigenesis induced by dimethylbenza(a)anthracene significantly inhibited tumor formation. "These data indicate that apigenin inhibited skin papillomas and showed the tendency to decrease conversion of papillomas to carcinomas."

SKULLCAP

Huang, H. C., H. R. Wang, and L. M. Hsieh. 1994. Antiproliferative effect of baicalein, a flavonoid from a Chinese herb, on vascular smooth muscle cell. *Eur. J. Pharmacol.* 4, 351:91–93.

Kimura, Y., N. Matsushita, and H. Okuda. 1997. Effects of baicalein isolated from *Scutellaria baicalensis* on interleukin 1 beta- and tumor necrosis factor alpha-induced adhesion molecule expression in cultured human umbilical vein endothelial cells. *J. Ethnopharmacol.* 57 (1):63–67.

Kimura, Y., H. Okuda, and Z. Ogita. 1997. Effects of flavonoids isolated from *Scuttellariae radix* on fibrinolytic system induced by trypsin in human umbilical vein endothelial cells. *J. Nat. Prod.* 60 (6):598–601.

Kimura, Y., K. Yokoi, N. Matsushita, and H. Okuda. 1997. Effects of flavonoids isolated from *scutellariae radix* on the production of tissue-type plasminogen activator and plasminogen activator inhibitor-1 induced by thrombin receptor agonist peptide in cultured human umbilical vein endothelial cells. *J. Pharm. Pharmacol.* 49 (8):816–22.

Lin, C. C., and D. E. Shieh. 1996. The anti-inflammatory activity of *Scutellaria rivularis* extracts and its active components, baicalin, baicalein and wogonin. *Am. J. Chin. Med.* 24 (1):31–36.

MacGregor, F. B., V. E. Abernathy, S. Dahabia, I. Cobden, and P. C. Hayes. 1989. *British Medical Journal* 299:1156–57.

Nagai, T., Y. Suzuki, T. Tomimori, and H. Yamada. 1995. Antiviral activity of plant flavonoid, 5,7,4'-trihydroxy-8-methoxyflavone, from the roots of *Scutellaria baicalensis* against influenza A (H3N2) and B viruses. *Biol. Pharm. Bull.* 18 (2):295–99.

Wood, H. C., and A. Osol. 1943. *The dispensary of the United States of America.* 23rd ed. Philadelphia: J. B. Lippincott.

Improve your mood, lose weight and curb your cravings, simply by learning the amazing...

SECRETS *of* SEROTONIN

CAROL HART

You don't need a prescription for it and you can't buy it at a drug store—that's because serotonin is a natural hormone that you already possess. Now, author Carol Hart tells you how to increase your serotonin levels through food, and exercise, and other natural ways to control your mood swings, your weight, food and alcohol cravings, and much more!

SECRETS OF SEROTONIN
Carol Hart
0-312-96087-5___$5.99 U.S.___$7.99 Can.

Research in herbs, natural supplements and longevity is accelerating. If you wish to keep up with the latest information in living longer and treating medical conditions naturally, subscribe to Dr. Ray Sahelian's *Longevity Research Update* newsletter. Dr. Sahelian will provide unbiased information that is bound to improve the quality of your life. There are no ads in this eight-page newsletter. All the facts are referenced with the latest journal articles.

Call (310) 821-2409 to order the newsletter or Dr. Sahelian's books (see his biography on the inside back cover for a list). You may also order by sending a check. Credit cards are accepted. Also see his website *www.raysahelian.com* for more information.

Name _____

Address _____

City/State Zip _____

Telephone _____ e-mail _____

4 issues of *Longevity Research Update* $16.00
8 issues of *Longevity Research Update* $28.00
16 issues of *Longevity Research Update* $48.00
Back issues are $1.00 each   _____
TOTAL   _____

The newsletter began in January 1996 and is published four times a year in January, April, July, and October.

Longevity Research Center
P.O. Box 12619
Marina Del Rey, CA 90295